SAFETY IN MEDICINE

Edited by

CHARLES VINCENT

University College London

and

BAS DE MOL

University of Amsterdam

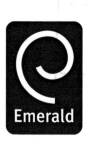

Emerald

United Kingdom – North America – Japan – India – Malaysia – China – Australasia

JAI Press is an imprint of Emerald Group Publishing Limited
Howard House, Wagon Lane, Bingley BD16 1WA, UK

First edition 2007

British Library Cataloguing in Publication Data
A catalogue record for this book is available from the British Library

ISBN: 978-0-08-043656-2

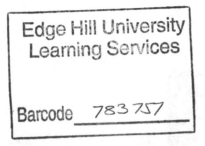

Certificate number ....1985........

Awarded in recognition of
Emerald's production
department's adherence to
quality systems and processes
when preparing scholarly
journals for print

INVESTOR IN PEOPLE

CONTENTS

vi

FOREWORD

NEW TECHNOLOGIES AND WORK – NETWORK
AN EXERCISE IN LONG-RANGE SCIENTIFIC INQUIRY

Bernhard Wilpert[1], *Berlin University of Technology, Berlin, Germany*

This volume presents the outcome from the 16th workshop of NeTWork in 1998. Its over-all theme was "Risk and Safety in Medicine" which extended the past focus of workshop themes into a new area. While in previous years high hazard industries were the main topics, this time the centre of interest became safety in medical services, particularly in operating theatres.

THE NATURE AND PURPOSE OF NETWORK

NeTWork is an international, interdisciplinary study group with the objective of advancing the study and intellectual penetration of social and scientific problems posed by the diffusion of modern technologies in all domains of work life. Over almost two decades NeTWork, partially supported by the Werner Reimers Foundation (Bad Homburg, Germany) and the Maison des Sciences de l'Homme (Paris), has held annual workshops relating to the overall theme of new technologies and work. These have covered a wide range of topics that included human error, training, distributed decision making and management (see appendix A).

While the original activities of NeTWork began with a wide coverage of subthemes, more recent preoccupations focused more specifically on a theme of great scientific and social significance:

safety of high technology systems and the role of human factors contributing to either breakdowns or the maintenance of hazardous systems.

---

[1] This paper is based on a previous draft by J. Reason and B. Wilpert

The past few years have seen a succession of major disasters afflicting a wide range of complex technologies: nuclear power plants, chemical installations, spacecraft, roll-on-roll-off ferries, commercial and military air craft, off-shore oil and gas platforms, telecommunication systems, computerised stock exchanges, high-tec medical services, hazardous goods transport and modern railway networks.

At a purely surface level, these accidents varied widely in their specific causes and consequences. At a more fundamental level, however, they shared a number of important features:

(a)   They occurred within well-defended systems that were proof against single failure, either human or mechanical.

(b)   They arose from the adverse conjunction of several distinct causal events. Moreover, a large proportion of these multiple causes were present within the system long before the accidents occurred.

(c)   The contribution of human factors rather than technical failures played a dominant role in all of these accidents.

A point has been reached in the development of technology where the greatest dangers stem from the insidious accumulation of latent or delayed action, i.e. human failures occurring primarily within the organisational, design and managerial sectors. The availability of cheap computing power has effected radical changes in the relationship between advanced technological systems and the people who control them:

(a)   Systems have become automated. In many new technologies, operators exercise remote supervisory control rather than direct, hands-on, manipulation of the process.

(b)   This control is centralised in the hands of a few individuals.

(c)   Systems have become larger, more complex and more dangerous: greater amounts of hazardous material are concentrated in single sites (chemical and nuclear power plants); there are more potential victims (advanced transport systems).

(d)   Elaborate 'defences-in-depth' make systems more opaque to the people who control them.

(e)   Flexible working conditions make it imperative that operators continuously explore the boundaries of their workspace in order to optimize various aspects of their performance. Yet the presence of automation and engineered safety systems obscures the boundaries between safe and unsafe operation.

We can trace four ages of safety concern. The first was the *technical age* in which the main focus was upon operational and engineering methods for combating hazards. Then came the *human error age* in which remedial efforts were directed at reducing both the occurrence and the consequences on unsafe acts committed by those at the immediate human-system interface. But over the past decade we have moved into a third age, the *socio-technical age*. In this, the present age, we recognise that the major residual safety problems do not belong exclusively to either the technical or the human domains. Rather, they emerge, from as yet little understood interactions between the technical, social and organisational aspects of the system. For the most part, the search for safer systems in this third age has concentrated upon identifying retrospectively those organisational features that contributed to major accidents such as Bhopal, Challenger, the 'Herald of Free Enterprise', Piper Alpha, King's Cross, Clapham Junction and Chernobyl. These case study analyses have yielded valuable insights into the organisational pathways by which fallible high-level decisions turn into the unsafe acts of those at the 'sharp end' of the system.

In highly regulated systems safety problems may also occur because of factors external to the organisation, such as regulation problems and dysfunctional relations between organisations, which herald an overlapping fourth age, *the inter-organisational age* in which efforts are also concentrated on the improvement of inter-organisational interactions.

Yet it is clear that investigations limited to accident-prone systems are not sufficient to identify those organisational characteristics which distinguish safe from unsafe systems. In order to meet the challenges of the socio-technical age and of the inter-organisational age, we need to seek out and describe the characteristics of high-reliability systems and their interactions. That is, organisations, operating in hazardous environments, that succeed in achieving a high degree of *relative* safety. In short: we need to define system health as well as system morbidity.

How NeTWork Works

The themes of annual workshops are planned and evaluated by a small 'core group' whose membership varies slightly according to the respective sub-theme to be treated. Two or three "godfathers" further detail a chosen sub-theme and propose a list of prospective participants. The choice of invitees is made internationally *ad personam* on the basis of their active research involvement with respect to the sub-theme or corresponding practice experience. Thus more than 160 persons from 20 countries participated in the NeTWork workshops between 1983 and 1999.

All contributions to a given workshop are distributed to all participants several weeks in advance in order to facilitate their thorough reading before the workshop itself. Only short statements are possible for each contributor summarising the main points of his/her paper contribution in order to maximise thorough discussion and proposals for the improvement of each contribution. The workshop's "godfathers" usually serve as editors for the preparation of the publication which is usually developed from each meeting. So far 13 publications have appeared from these NeTWork activities (see appendix B). Three more are in preparation. The model of this international and interdisciplinary exchange has meanwhile been adopted by various other institutions.

The administration of NeTWork activities is managed by staff of the Berlin University of Technology, Institute of Psychology - Research Center Systems Safety: Prof. Bernhard Wilpert (Speaker) and Babette Fahlbruch (previously: Prof. Antonio Ruiz Quintanilla and Matthias Freitag, Workshop Coordinators). The Werner Reimers Foundation and the Maison des Sciences de l'Homme lend further administrative and material support.

Today, the participants in NeTWork form an international, interdisciplinary network of professionals which world-wide seeks its equal in terms of its unique and productive mix: philosophers, historians, engineers, management experts, sociologists, psychologists, physiologists, physicians, economists, ergonomists united in a common concern for the improvement of safety and reliability of complex modern socio-technical systems.

SUMMARY

Close to two decades of successful theme oriented cooperation of a large international, interdisciplinary group consisting of internationally reputed as well as young promising scholars and experienced practitioners is in itself a remarkable achievement. This was only possible on the basis of the unbureaucratic support from two enlightened institutions devoted to the furthering of national and international cooperation among human sciences: the Werner Reimers Foundation (Bad Homburg) and the Maison des Sciences de l'Homme (Paris).

APPENDICES

NeTWork Workshop Themes

1983   New Information Technologies and Work

1984   New Technology and Human Error

1985   Changing Work Structures and Work Meanings in the Context of New Information Technologies

1986   Information Technology, Competence, and Employment

1987   What and How to Teach in Information Technology

1988   Modeling Distributed Decision Making

1989   Telematics and Work

1990   Managing New Technologies

1991   Control of Safety

1992   Growth, Change, and Industrial Safety

1993   The Use of Rules to Achieve Safety

1994   In Search of Safety

1995   Theories and Methods of Event Analysis

1996   The Organization-Safety Link

1997   Coping with Accelerating Technologies

1998   Risk and Safety in Medicine

1999   Achieving Successful Safety Interventions

NeTWork Publications

Jens Rasmussen, Keith Duncan and Jacques Leplat (eds.), (1987). *New Technology and Human Error*. Chichester: Wiley.

Véronique de Keyser, Thoralf Qvale, Bernhard Wilpert, & S. Antonio Ruiz Quintanilla (eds.), (1988). *The Meaning of Working and Technological Options*. Chichester: Wiley.

Lisanne Bainbridge and S. Antonio Ruiz Quintanilla (Eds.), (1989). *Developing Skills with Information Technology*. Chichester: Wiley.

Malcolm Warner, Werner Wobbe and Peter Brödner (Eds.), (1989). *New Technology and Manufacturing Management. Strategic Choices for Flexible Production Systems*. Chichester: Wiley.

Jens Rasmussen, Berndt Brehmer and Jacques Leplat (Eds.), (1990). *Distributed Decision Making. Cognitive Models for Complex Work Environments*. Chichester: Wiley.

Robert A. Roe and Erik Andriessen (Eds.), (1994). *Telematics and Work*. Hove: Lawrence Erlbaum.

Bernhard Wilpert and Thoralf Qvale (Eds.), (1993). *Reliability and Safety in Hazardous Work Systems - Approaches to Analysis and Design*. Hove: Lawrence Erlbaum.

Andriessen, J.H.E. and Roe, R.A. (Eds.), (1994). *Telematics and Work*. Hove: Lawrence Erlbaum.

Hale, A, Freitag, M. and Wilpert, B. (Eds.), (1997). *After the Event - From Accident to Organizational Learning*. Oxford: Pergamon.

Hale, A. and Baram, M. (Eds.) (1998) *Safety Management and the Challenge of Organisational Change*. Oxford: Pergamon.

Vincent, C. and de Mol, B. (Eds.) *Safety in Medicine*. Oxford: Pergamon.

Furthermore, based on NeTWork-workshops two special issues have been published in learned journals:

Maurice de Montmollin (ed.), (1990). Skills, Qualifications, Employment. *Applied Psychology*, Vol. 39 (2)

Jaques Leplat and Andrew Hale (eds.), (1998). Safety Rules. Safety Science, Vol. 29 (3).

INTRODUCTION

Charles Vincent, Department of Psychology, University College London, London, UK.
Bas de Mol, Department of Cardio-thoracic Surgery, University of Amsterdam, The Netherlands.

The recent report of the National Patient Safety Foundation at the American Medical Association begins with a splendid and apposite quote from Charles Dickens.

> "It was the best of times, it was the worst of times, it was the age of wisdom, it was the age of foolishness, it was the epoch of belief, it was the epoch of disbelief ...".

The authors go on to say that:

> "For health care at the end of the twentieth century, it is also the best of times and the worst of times, a time of paradoxes and contrasts. On the one hand, splendid new knowledge, more finely honed skills, and technical advances bring sophisticated treatments to larger and more fragile populations of people than ever before. On the other hand, media and public attention is focussed on medical accidents – chemotherapy overdoses, wrong limb surgery catastrophic missed diagnoses. Stunning success and appalling failure are arrayed in contrast to each other. It is in this setting that discussions about patient safety are now taking place" (Cook *et al.*, 1998).

The conference on which this book is based brought together safety researchers and practitioners from high technology industries and healthcare researchers and clinicians. The purpose of the conference, and this book, was to explore the differences and parallels between safety in healthcare and in other domains. Before we discuss the structure of the book, we will introduce some of the problems facing those working in advanced healthcare systems, which form the backdrop to any discussion of safety in medicine.

Public Expectations and Risk Communication

Disease itself, so much a part of life in previous centuries, is for many adults now an exceptional event in an otherwise safe and well-ordered life. The general public now have high expectations of healthcare, as they do of other industries and services. People expect to emerge safely from hospital, just as they expect to arrive safely after a flight on a commercial airline. The fate of being injured, rather than saved, by modern healthcare can be experienced as a terrible injustice. There are of course some major differences between safety management in health and that in aviation and industry. Most importantly, disease and death are acceptable, although unwanted, outcomes of good healthcare. It is therefore much more difficult to identify the contribution of poor healthcare in the final outcome. Harm to a patient may simply be a complication of treatment, although in many cases unsafe practice cannot be excluded as a contributory cause.

All clinicians understand that risk is at the heart of all medical practice. Every decision is a balance of risks and benefits, but it is not always easy to convey this to the patient and their relatives. Even when there is some knowledge of the general risks associated with a treatment, it may be impossible to say what the risks are for that particular patient. A further problem is that the balance of risks and benefits is different in the short and long term. For instance, with an elective, preventive procedure (e.g. heart valve replacement, carotid endarterectomy) there is an immediate increased risk of operative mortality, but a long term reduction in the risks of mortality or disability in the future (Lloyd *et al.*, 1999; Rothwell and Warlow, 1999).

The medico-legal environment also complicates matters both for patients and clinicians. For instance, in The Netherlands, doctors have the duty to inform patients not only about the risks of a specific medical treatment but also about possible alternatives. A Dutch court recently judged that this includes the obligation to inform patients about the availability of other hospitals where better monitoring facilities are available that reduce the risk of neurological damage during scoliosis correction surgery. So, hospitals must ensure that they stay well informed about each other's technical possibilities, strengths and weaknesses.

Lack of acceptance or understanding of the risks inherent in medical procedures underlies some of the feelings of injustice experienced by patients whose disease does not respond satisfactorily to treatment. On occasion, claims for compensation are made solely because of poor understanding of the risks involved. In other instances, however, injuries are clearly due to problems within the healthcare system. Adverse outcome may be due to human error, shortcomings of an organisation, breakdown of equipment or a device, inferior practice and violation of protocols and accepted standards of practice. For instance, a series of mishaps with drugs and devices have caused public outrage, resulting in compensation settlements between patients and health authorities and manufacturers (Birchard, 1999; de Mol and Fielder 1997; Sandman, 1991).

For all the high profile media reports, litigation after adverse outcomes is surprisingly infrequent. In the Harvard Medical Practice Study, the ratio of adverse events due to substandard care to paid claims was sixteen to one (Localio *et al.*, 1991). The number of claims is only the tip of the iceberg when it comes to estimating the suffering and the extent of personal injury due to avoidable adverse events. Poor communication between patient and health workers aggravates the patient's and relatives' perception of injustice, this being an important contributing factor in litigation (Vincent *et al.*, 1994). Studies on specialist obstetric practices have shown that poor communication, rather than poor skills, determine the probability of recurrent medicolegal actions against a doctor (Hickson *et al.*, 1994; Bovbjerg and Petronis, 1994). Full disclosure of risks and good communication are fundamental to the clinician-patient relationship and to the avoidance of litigation. More cynically it can be suggested that poor medical practices can be concealed by risk avoidance, risk sharing and good manners, wrapped in a glossy attentive environment. This is a risk management strategy of a kind, but not what we mean by risk management. When we talk about risk and safety management, understanding and intervention have to begin at the level of the care and interventional process itself.

Safety Management in Healthcare

Risk management may be defined as "the process of making and carrying out decisions to minimise adverse effects and accidental losses. Making these decisions requires identification, analysis, choice, implementation, and monitoring with regard to risks" (Bignell, 1984).

When discussing risk to patients, the assessment may be related to a therapeutic or diagnostic intervention, which in turn may be just a step in the process to improve health or the key procedure finally determining outcome. A safety assessment may concern a task, procedure, or process, or may be a feature of the performance of a drug or device. When we look at an industrial process in order to assess and manage its safety, five aspects can be taken into consideration (Perrow, 1987; Laffel and Blumenthal, 1989):

- the chances of failure of the system as a whole or of its various subsystems
- the failure modes and scenarios
- setting a safety standard and maintaining and/or resetting norms of safety
- the potential or real damage related to the failure
- damage control, compensation, and preventive measures

In healthcare and other domains, both commercial and societal interests determine which resource will be allocated to maintain safe practice. Safety is an explicit test for quality, and adverse outcome is often publicly depicted as a disaster either for workers or for the public in general. In healthcare, safety is an implicit duty of the workers and the organisation, which is rarely questioned by the healthcare professionals and managers themselves, by the public, or the supporting authorities. Some paramedics and doctors like to compare their jobs, the technical support systems they use, and their organisation with those of technologically sophisticated and high-risk activities, such as flying an aircraft or controlling a complex chemical process. While this may be true of some specialties and some people, the culture of healthcare is sometimes more akin to military and emergency services. While aviation, in commercial settings, is highly procedural, healthcare may be more akin to the unpredictable environment of military aviation. In these settings personal skills, endurance and a successful record of coping well with risks prove mastery. If danger threatens, the professional in charge feels justified in deviating from the protocol. Senior staff have great personal power, as the unsurpassed rulers of the working floor, to overrule decisions of juniors without being seriously questioned: they are free to apply unusual and unproven interventions simply with an appeal to their expert status.

In medicine, analysis of the phenomenon of adverse outcome has a multi-disciplinary character. Although these elements may vary, any analysis has to be based on observations at the individual level of the patient-doctor relationship, the organisational level dealing with the duties of institutional and professional bodies, the sector level in which the various streams of healthcare are assessed and compared, and the societal level at which policy making with respect to the funding of quality assurance of healthcare, claim behaviour of patients, and public risk perception are controlled.

This multidisciplinary perspective is still unusual in medicine, though there are examples of links being made between disciplines when tackling safety issues in healthcare. For instance, when confronted with implant failure of abdominal aortic endovascular grafts, the Dutch Society of Vascular Surgery and the Association for Intervention Radiology founded a multidisciplinary working group to promote the quality of the endovascular use of endoprostheses in the treatment of abdominal aneurysms. The working group recommended the introduction of a safety committee. This committee collects information from researchers and manufacturers, helps doctors to control and solve problems, and acts as an advisor to the Health Care Inspectorate. The indications for doing an endarterectomy of the carotid artery have now been linked to observed risks of mortality and morbidity in a specific hospital, as has the experience of supervising surgeons in seemingly simple operations such as below-the-knee amputations. The committee's multidisciplinary approach may also be useful for other professions that use 'critical' products like blood products, breast implants, or home laboratories for patients on anticoagulants.

Risk and Safety in Medicine: the NeTWork Conference

Previous NeTWork conferences (see the Foreword by Bernhard Wilpert) had addressed the subject of safety in a number of domains, but this was the first specifically concerned with healthcare. The proposal stressed the major problem of iatrogenic injury (harm to patients caused by treatment) and the growing interest in human factors approaches within medicine. Crude views of human error were being challenged by more sophisticated approaches developed in such fields as aviation, chemical and nuclear industries. Within this broad context, the role of new technologies was given particular attention as providing the potential both for enhancing safety and creating new risks.

Nineteen participants from a wide variety of disciplines and backgrounds attended the conference. Three were clinicians committed to human factors approaches, and others had experience of healthcare either as clinicians or researchers. Participants brought expertise from several domains and disciplines, but some had little experience of healthcare settings. Contributors with a medical background compared their experiences with those in other, industrial, sectors. The overwhelming response, both at the end of the meeting and in subsequent e-mail correspondence, was that this was a valuable and productive meeting.

Although we do not want to anticipate the contents of the chapters, especially the overview by Andrew Hale, a few points can be made about the meeting. First, there was remarkable recognition of common problems, for instance in the area of incident reporting and analysis, across different domains. However, the huge variability in modes of practice within medicine means that parallels may be drawn with a number of different domains: anaesthesia with aviation; accident and emergency medicine with military operations; and the hospital organisation as a whole with high risk business ventures. It is vital to choose appropriate reference groups when endeavouring to apply lessons across cultures and domains and to develop a good understanding of the structure, function and culture of each domain. It was clear to everyone present that there was huge scope for continuing development and application of approaches to safety throughout medicine. It was equally clear that the current pressure to develop and apply methods of reducing risk might come at the expense of sustained development and evaluation of methods of assessment and intervention.

There was also agreement between participants about the need to consider safety in a very wide context. For instance, there is concern that the increasing standardisation of medical practice, imposed through managed care in the United States, is a potential source of patient risk. This broad perspective was also apparent in the tentative conclusions reached about improving safety. Rather than the retraining or disciplining of individuals, the primary focus should be on organisational learning as the key to improving medical safety, both within and between organisations, in the form of sharing of knowledge and best practice. There is a multitude of unresolved problems in all domains, some being common to all areas.

For instance, the progressive 'shrinkage of validity' with successive analyses of incidents, advantages and disadvantages of different approaches to incident reporting, how to conduct valid and useful analyses of large numbers of events, how to produce feedback and, eventually, organisational learning.

Structure of the Book

We originally envisaged this book as dividing into four distinct sections covering, respectively, the conceptual foundations of safety management, approaches to investigating the nature and frequency of problems, analyses of the causes of adverse outcomes and risk to patients and, finally, approaches to improving safety and reducing risk.   As the chapters arrived, however, it became clear that this formal structure was not workable and not, in fact, necessary.   While chapters differed in emphasis, almost all were concerned with all four aspects of safety management. The chapters are therefore simply ordered to accord with their principal emphasis, beginning with conceptual foundations and moving towards safety management.

The first chapter gives an overview of approaches to safety in the psychological and organisational literature (Fahlbruch, Wilpert and Vincent) and provides essential background information for readers who may not be familiar with the safety literature. Jens Rasmussen then tackles the vexed question of the nature of human error and its role in healthcare, arguing for greater sophistication in our understanding of error and for a broad multi-faceted understanding of safety. Anne-Sophie Nyssen's analysis of human error in anaesthesia, and her description of the anaesthetic work process, then underlines the complexity of the clinical environment and the need for a subtle and careful analysis of clinical decisions and their consequences.

Safety researchers and practitioners in most domains have made use of accident data and analyses of near misses as a route to improving safety. Three papers address this theme in relation to healthcare. Sven Staender and colleagues describe incident reporting systems in anaesthesia while Sue Bogner and Sally Taylor-Adams describe formal approaches to the analysis of incidents in healthcare which draw on human factors and systems methodologies. Such analyses point to the range of human and organisational influences on safety in healthcare, which are addressed directly in the next three papers.   Jane Carthey and colleagues report an ambitious and innovative study of human and organisational factors in cardiac surgery; Stephan Marsch reports a programme to develop team performance in anaesthesia and surgery; André Büssing shows how the fundamental structure of healthcare organisations can be investigated in relation to their impact on the quality and safety of healthcare.

Previous chapters emphasised the need to take a very broad organisational view of safety. The next chapters demonstrate the need to take a long, temporal perspective. Manon Cromheecke and colleagues, in a persuasive analysis of failures of heart valves, show that while fundamental design faults were the root of the problem, failures of regulation and management of these problems were evident over many years in a number of organisations. Fred van den Anker and Udo Voges then show, in different ways, how such problems may be anticipated by careful and intelligent preparation and by the application of systematic approaches to the introduction of new technologies in healthcare. Finally, two chapters reflect on the nature of safety management and its particular application in healthcare. Michael Baram draws lessons from the chemical industry's approach to regulation and Andrew Hale provides an overview of both the conference and the chapters themselves, examining key themes that emerged and identifying the main challenges for future research and practice in healthcare

A Final Word

All the authors deserve a vote of thanks from the editors for their patience with the editing process and willingness to respond to requests. In the final stages Maria Woloshynowych, Sally Taylor-Adams and Laura Seymour read all the chapters and made many improvements and corrections. Most important of all, Pam La Rose bravely tackled the Herculean task of producing a camera ready book with all her usual attention to detail and good humour. Without her care and patience there would be no book.

REFERENCES

Bignell V., J. Fortune (1984). *Understanding system failures*. Manchester University Press, Manchester.

Birchard K. (1999). Irish hepatitis C compensation ruling. *Lancet*, **353**, 1507.

Bovbjerg R. R. and K. R. Petronis (1994). The relationship between physicians' malpractice claims history and later claims. *Journal of the American Medical Association*, **272**, 1421-1426.

Cook R. I., D. D. Woods and C. Miller (1998). *A tale of two stories: contrasting view of patient safety*. National Patient Safety Foundation, American Medical Association.

de Mol B. A. and J. H. Fielder (1997). Systemic accident analysis of deaths due to failed Björk-Shiley heart valves. *International Journal of Risk and Safety in Medicine*, **10**, 243-247.

Hickson G. B, E. W. Clayton, S. S. Entman, C. S. Miller, P. B. Githens, K. Whetten-Goldstein and F. A. Sloan (1994). Obstetricians' prior malpractice experience and patients' satisfaction with care. *Journal of the American Medical Association*, **272**, 1583-1587.

Laffel G. and D. Blumenthal (1989). The case for using industrial quality management science in health care organisations. *Journal of the American Medical Association*, **262**, 2869-2873.

Lloyd A. J., P. D. Hayes, N. J. M. London, P. R. F. Bell and A. R. Naylor (1999). Patients' ability to recall risk associated with treatment options. *Lancet*, **353**, 645-646.

Localio A. R., A. G. Lawthers, T. A. Brennan, N. M. Laird, L. E. Herbert, L. M. Petersen, J. P. Newhouse, P. C. Weiler and H. H. Hiatt (1991). Relation between malpractice claims and adverse events due to negligence. Results of the Harvard Malpractice Study III. *New England Journal of Medicine*, **325**, 245-251.

Perrow Ch. (1987.) *Normal accidents. Living with high-risk technologies*. Basic Book Publ Inc., New York.

Rothwell P. M. and C. P. Warlow (1999). Interpretation of operative risks of individual surgeons. The European Carotid Surgery Trialists' Collaborative Group. *Lancet*, **353**, 1325.

Sandman P. M. (1991). Emerging communication responsibilities of epidemiologists. *Journal of Clinical Epidemiology*, **44**(suppl. 1), 41S-45S.

Vincent C., M. Young and A. Philips (1994). Why do people sue doctors? A study of patients and relatives taking legal action. *Lancet*, **343**, 1609-1613.

CHAPTER 1

APPROACHES TO SAFETY

Babette Fahlbruch, Bernhard Wilpert, University of Technology, Berlin, Germany
Charles Vincent, University College London, London, UK.

INTRODUCTION

The safety of patients in hospital has always been an absolute priority of individual clinicians, being enshrined in the Hippocratic Oath as 'First, do no harm'. However, while the monitoring of medical care can be traced back to the early 20th Century, systematic attempts to assess the quality of care have only become widespread in the last 20 years. The quality of care encompasses, in one influential definition, six dimensions of effectiveness, efficiency, appropriateness, acceptability, access to care and equity (Maxwell, 1984). Arguably safety is encompassed in these dimensions but, in practice, the specific study of adverse outcomes for patients has not been the overriding priority (Vincent, 1997). In some countries, such as Canada, attempts to improve quality and safety have gone hand in hand. In Britain, attempts to improve safety, in the form of risk management, have been driven by a rise in litigation and developed separately from quality initiatives. Only now, with the advent of clinical governance, are quality and safety initiatives being integrated.

Approaches to quality include a bewildering number of terms and definitions. One author identified twenty-six separate approaches to quality improvement in medicine (Taylor, 1996), though many are similar in both aim and content. Quality assurance tends to be associated with external inspection and accreditation. Quality improvement usually refers to internal reviews of the process of care, sometimes associated with the Total Quality Management approaches developed in industry. In Britain quality has been most associated with clinical audit, a cycle of activities involving the measurement of care, comparison with a standard of some kind (whether process or outcome) and, ideally, interventions to improve quality where necessary. Most reliance is placed, in clinical audit and elsewhere in medicine, on large scale sampling. While case histories have an honourable tradition clinically, they are distrusted in research and audit.

There are few equivalents, thus far, of accident investigation in which a single incident is examined in detail.

While there have been a number of attempts to learn from approaches to quality taken in industry and elsewhere, comparatively little attention has been paid to approaches to safety in other domains. Psychologists who work in medicine are primarily concerned with the psychology of health and illness, rather than with the practice of medicine (with some exceptions such as medical decision making). Conversely, safety researchers and practitioners in other domains have been little involved in medicine. Only in the last few years have clinicians and researchers in medicine begun to consider human factors, ergonomics and the psychology of safety as topics that might have something to contribute in the medical arena. Approaches to quality in medicine have, by and large, not drawn on psychology. There has been little attention, for instance, to psychological approaches to error, organisational behaviour, safety culture, and other topics that would be considered basic to safety in other domains.

In the context of the book this chapter introduces some of the main approaches to safety taken in other areas, selecting those that seem to have most to offer medicine. The purpose of this chapter is to set the scene for the chapters that follow, in which these approaches are applied in a variety of clinical settings.

PSYCHOLOGICAL APPROACHES TO SAFETY

Traditionally, psychology has viewed safety as 'occupational safety'. The focus was on the individual worker and his/her personality, motivation and competence in the workplace. The study of safety primarily concerned the investigation of human error and its causes. Early psychological human error classification attempts (e.g. Weimer, 1922) as well as their more recent successors (Norman, 1981; Rasmussen 1987; Reason, 1990a) all viewed human errors as the results of actions which deviate from the intended goals due to individual dispositional factors. These different approaches reflect the scope of traditional occupational safety and can be summarised under the 'person model' (Reason, 1995) in which emphasis is put on human error, unsafe acts and personal injuries.

In the last few years the focus has shifted from personal characteristics to the influence of work place to organisational factors (Sheehy and Chapman, 1987). Prevention of occupational accidents and safeguarding of employee health, as well as protection of environment, have become critical elements within a holistic framework of comprehensive 'integrated safety management' strategies (Zimolong, 1996). Hoyos and Ruppert (1993) even use the term 'system safety' as a key-term for this 'new perspective'. Attention is directed to the encompassing organisational system as well as the individual workers and their work places. Intervention mainly aims at designing safer workplaces. The 'person model' and the 'engineering model' are therefore still the main paradigms of analysis and intervention.

Although this present-day approach to occupational safety also addresses the organisation and management, it still falls short of the notion of total system breakdown or 'systems disasters' (Reason, 1990a). System disasters are characterised by accidents due to a loss of control of large scale, low risk – high hazard organisations with drastic negative consequences for people and environment. Examples of such accidents are cases in which high concentrations of energy or toxic materials break their barriers, with dramatic, traumatic and extremely costly consequences. The context for these events is usually a large scale socio-technical system with high hazard potential. It is this domain of high hazard organisations and their potential for disastrous breakdowns that Fahlbruch and Wilpert (1999) reserved the notion of 'system safety'. In line with Roland and Moriarty (1990), they define "system safety as a quality of a system that allows the system to function without major breakdowns under predetermined conditions with an acceptable minimum of accidental loss and unintended harm to the organisation and its environment" (Fahlbruch and Wilpert, 1999).

The remainder of this chapter is structured in three parts. The first part addresses the growing phenomenon of large and complex socio-technical systems with high hazard potential, which both clinicians and researchers have argued have important similarities to medicine (Reason, 1995; Leape, 1994). The second part groups and discusses a selection of relevant literature under the hitherto developed main theoretical paradigms. In a final section we consider one particular theoretical perspective of particular importance to medicine.

LARGE AND COMPLEX SOCIO-TECHNICAL SYSTEMS

In the 20th century the development and spread of a new category of technical installations and systems arose whose sheer size and complexity outscored everything known in the past (La Porte, 1994). With the increase in complexity came a corresponding increase in the potential for hazards, particularly in unforgiving environments such as civil and military aviation, high-speed earth-bound traffic, off-shore oil drilling, nuclear power production and chemical process plants. To the list we can now add medicine, because of its increasing complexity and technological sophistication. The typical characteristics of such highly complex systems - variably labelled as high risk or high hazard - are "high potential consequences, tight functional coupling (see below) and potentially rapid evolution of untoward events" (Rochlin, 1993). Prime importance is given to failure avoidance and effective production process and service control in such systems. Case studies of many industrial disasters convincingly demonstrate that system breakdowns are more than simply the result of operator error or the failure of a technical component. They are due to a combination of interdependent factors from various systems levels such as technical, individual, work team, supervision and management, organisational features and extra-organisational environment. In this realisation lies the logic of the 'defence-in-depth-design' of such systems: one single factor alone will not cause a major accident.

According to Fahlbruch and Wilpert (1999), it is curious that organisational science and psychology have for a long time neglected the study of hazardous systems while at the same time the number of these systems is increasing world-wide (Roberts, 1992). To conceive, design, construct, run, and maintain large scale technical installations was initially seen as almost exclusively the province of engineers. However, two particular factors have brought psychology irrevocably into the picture: recent industrial catastrophes and social value change. First, the re-analysis of major accidents such as Seveso, Bhopal, Three Mile Island, Exxon Valdez and Chernobyl convincingly demonstrated that it was the interaction of individual errors and poor decisions with managerial, organisational and extra-organisational factors which determined the events. Secondly large sections of the population were directly affected by the consequences of the catastrophes, both physically and psychologically. The growth of green and environmental movements has also contributed to a heightened public perception of these objectively existing hazards. The perceived uncontrollability of these risks may have kindled further concern. Based on the experience of industrial catastrophes and the given social context, the combined forces of engineering, organisational, political and psychological sciences facilitated new theorising and the development of more adequate models of the generation of systems accidents (see below).

BASIC PARADIGMS AND THEIR PSYCHOLOGICAL IMPLICATIONS

By basic paradigms we mean the various research strands which take up different perspectives or starting points. The paradigms discussed below represent the dominant ones in the field of system safety. They vary in their theoretical sophistication and in their potential to offer practice relevant recommendations.

The Pessimistic View

Perrow's 'normal accident theory' maintains that serious accidents are an unavoidable 'normal' aspect of high hazard systems due to their intrinsic characteristics of to dimensions: 'interactive complexity' and 'tight- coupling'. Interactive complexity is characterised by interactions of system components which are unforeseen by designers, unfamiliar, unplanned and difficult to understand for operators. It is contrasted to directly understood, familiar and expected interactions so called 'linear interactions' (Perrow, 1984). In contrast, tight-coupling means that the system processes are highly time dependent and invariant, in the sense that everything happens comparatively fast and production processes follow specific invariant sequences. Both factors result in limited resources and constrained opportunities for recovery if something goes wrong. Potential hazards must usually be mitigated by preplanned safety devices and protective design features.

The combination of both, high interactive complexity and tight-coupling, leads to the explosive mix which, according to the normal accident theory, will eventually and inevitably result in major system failures, in accidents and catastrophes of installations. The true danger of these systems lies in their inherent potential for hazards and in the systems themselves and not in the failure of their components and their operators. According to Perrow, the only rational political option should be to ban and to give up technologies with high catastrophe potential, such as nuclear weaponry and nuclear power production installations (and presumably also space flights with nuclear reactors aboard). With this perspective the role of psychology seems to be restricted to risk communication in the sense that it ought to alert the public to the true dangers of such high hazard systems. Some systems within medicine are certainly characterised by interactive complexity and 'tight-coupling', as a number of chapters in this book demonstrate. Cardiac surgery, for instance, requires complex interaction between people and is, while sequences are far from invariant, time is critical and there may be very limited opportunity for recovery in the event of a problem (see Carthey, chapter 7).

Sagan analysed all available evidence of near accidents of the system of Strategic Air Command (SAC) of the United States in peacetime and crisis situations in the 60's and 70's and concludes that his analyses support the assumptions of the normal accident theory although "there has never been an accidental nuclear detonation, there have been numerous close calls with US nuclear weapons" (Sagan, 1993). Sagan's keen analyses of the tremendous technical and organisational complexity and interactions of SAC operations convincingly shows the theoretical and practical usefulness of organisational and psychological approaches to the understanding of safety and reliability of complex high hazard systems. Similar demonstrations of the often complex interactions of technical, social and organisational factors on all system levels in producing (near-) accidents are seen in analyses of (near-)accidents in nuclear power plants (Reason, 1990a; Wilpert and Klumb, 1991), of managerial contributions to accidents (Brascamp *et al.*, 1993), and the re-analyses of the Challenger disaster (Starbuck and Millikan, 1988; Heimann, 1993; Vaughan, 1996), although their authors may not necessarily be counted as adherents of the normal accident theory.

The Optimistic View

In contrast to the pessimistic 'normal accident' tradition, the interdisciplinary research group of the University of California at Berkeley studies 'High Reliability Organisations – HRO', organisations which "continue to exist, to adapt, and to perform superbly in defiance of traditional analysis" (Rochlin, 1993). As examples of HROs the Berkley Group investigated air traffic control, electric utility grid management and nuclear power plants as well as US Navy aircraft carriers. Their research explicitly aims at explicating the factors that contribute to the extraordinarily reliable, often near peak performance of such systems (La Porte and Metlay, 1996).

According to the findings of the Berkeley Group (La Porte and Metlay, 1996), HROs' internal processes and external relationships are characterised by

- a strong sense of mission and operational goals,
- high technical competence and operational performance,
- structural flexibility and redundancy,
- next to hierarchical authority patterns also collegial ones with flexible decision making,
- continual search for improvement through experience feedback,
- reward structures for the discovery and reporting of error,
- an organisational culture of reliability.

External relationships are of particular importance for HROs. The problem of public trust and confidence in such institutions becomes ever more urgent because the number of large scale technical systems grows, and with it the number of high hazard systems. To have or not to have public trust and confidence may in many cases be for HROs a question of survival or death. Many high hazard organisations are facing the difficult task of maintaining or even recapturing public trust which has been lost. The latter problem is even more difficult to solve than the former one, due to the 'asymmetry principle': "When it comes to winning trust, the playing field is not level. It is tilted toward distrust" (Slovic, 1993). This is of particular importance in healthcare. In Britain, the USA, Australia and elsewhere a number of high-profile disasters have severely shaken public confidence in medicine and the regaining of trust is of paramount importance.

Research on HROs encompasses a wide range of fundamental safety issues such as leadership and goal setting, organisational design and governance, personnel attitudes and norms, incentive systems, and inter-organisational relations and communication. For instance, Roberts (1990) describes the results of an in-depth case study of two nuclear powered air craft carriers and neatly illustrates the various organisational and managerial strategies to cope with the problems of high complexity and tight coupling (Perrow, 1984), as well as the personnel characteristics of staff considered as relevant to safety (Shrivastava, 1987): good training, high motivation and adequate personnel. The dynamics of decision making in HROs are found to be subject to frequent changes and fluctuating across hierarchical levels according to situational demands, which seems to contradict some received decision making theories (Roberts, 1992; Roberts *et al.*, 1994). As yet there are no HRO studies of healthcare, although clinicians might well endorse many of the HRO factors as being characteristic of high performance teams. The

HRO perspective seems a potentially very fruitful approach to examining the factors that distinguish healthcare teams and organisations.

The Safety Cultural View

The term 'organisational culture' is, broadly speaking, used in two senses. The concept may denote the mental, cognitive and emotional features of its members (Turner, 1978; Schein, 1985) or it may refer to behaviour patterns and directly observable characteristics of a given collective (Mitroff *et al.*, 1989; Sackmann, 1983).

In matters of systems safety, we prefer a definition that encompasses behaviour. The 'working definition' of the British Advisory Committee on the Safety of Nuclear Installations is as follows:

"The safety culture of an organization is the product of individual and group values, attitudes, perceptions, competencies, and patterns of behavior that determine the commitment to, and the style and proficiency of, an organization's health and safety management" (ACSNI, 1993).

Wilpert (1991) argues that safety culture must be thought of in terms of 'the total system'. We need to transcend the traditional limitations of an exclusive focus on a single organisation, such as a nuclear power plant, and to consider all factors that are able to contribute to safety. We are dealing here with an inter-organisational phenomenon. We should therefore include important reference organisations, consulting bodies, regulators and public stakeholders. In healthcare this would imply that we should look beyond the hospital to the external environment, taking into account insurance companies, managed care organisations, government policies and so on. The concept of safety culture has stimulated theorising and empirical research by directing the attention to wider managerial, organisational, and inter-organisational issues of safety than has been the tradition of safety science, with its emphasis on human (operator) error like in the person model (Reason, 1995). Cases in point are the various attempts to operationalise and measure safety culture, to which we turn now.

Büttner (1997) systematically compares eight methodological approaches to the study of safety culture and evaluates them with reference to six evaluative dimensions used in the context of an analytic approach called 'Safety through Organizational Learning – SOL' (Wilpert *et al.*, 1994): standardisation, validity, reliability, objectivity, economy, practicability. The first five approaches thematise safety related attitudes and norms. An example of this is the Questionnaire of Employee Attitudes to Safety (Cox and Cox, 1991), which refers to safety culture as reflecting "the attitudes, beliefs, perceptions and values that employees share in relation to safety" (Cox and

Cox, 1991). The questionnaire consists of both standardised and open questions and was applied in European subsidiaries of a natural gas producing and distributing multinational company. The authors derive an empirical model of safety related attitude interactions based on factor analyses of their data.

The other three approaches broaden their remit to include behavioural and organisational variables. For example, the International Atomic Energy Agency (IAEA) developed Guidelines for the Assessment of Safety Culture in Organization Teams (ASCOT) for use in safety audits in nuclear power plants. The ASCOT-Guidelines assume that the essential characteristics of safety culture are commitment to safety on three levels (government and regulators, management and individual level). Data gathering is conducted by the method of open interviews on the basis of an ASCOT indicator list, document analysis and site visits.

The comparison of different analysis methods of safety culture and climate (Büttner, 1997) shows that different culture concepts lead to different operationalisations. Most of the methods are of a more exploratory character and further validation seems necessary. Nevertheless, the richness of ongoing research gives hope for improved methodological refinements and theoretical underpinnings. As yet there are, to our knowledge, no examinations of safety culture in healthcare, but once again this would mean a potentially fruitful research area.

Safety Management

Safety management is perhaps the most influential of the paradigms discussed, judging from the number of publications. A large variety of approaches have been developed in applied settings. In this section we illustrate some of the different research lines and approaches to safety management in the industrial field.

Reviews of the research literature on safety management suggest that the goal is mainly to identify factors that have influenced the safety performance of an organisation (Hale *et al.*, 1997). Publications include comparisons of companies with high and low accident rates (Haber *et al.*, 1990; Nichols and Marcus, 1990), case studies of high reliability organisations (Rochlin, 1989; Roberts, 1990), and investigations of major accidents (Groeneweg, 1992; Reason, 1990b; Wilpert and Klumb, 1991). Other authors focus on safety information systems (Kjellén, 1982) or on internal control systems (Hovden and Tinmannisvik, 1990; Hovden, 1996). According to Hale *et al.* (1997), only in the nuclear field are there explicit models of safety management systems modelling either key behaviours or levels of safety organisations (INSAG, 1991). Hale *et al.* (1997) proposed a framework for a safety management system including the concepts of problem solving cycles (Hale, 1985), levels of decision making (Reason, 1990a), risks as deviations and the life cycle. These concepts are modelled according to input, resources, transformation, output and control.

Rasmussen (1991a) discusses safety management as a problem of safety control on a more abstract level. For him, safety is managed by three different control strategies:

A reactive *feedback strategy,* used for distributed sources of low hazards, which aims to control safety empirically by ongoing measurements according to a certain acceptable level of safety, operationalised in accident or injury rates. This strategy is referred to as *empirical control by objective.* Methods are oriented to past events, such as event analyses, case studies and epidemiological approaches

A *feedforward strategy,* used for high hazard systems in rapid change, aims to control safety by proper design and operation, taking into account mechanisms underlying the system hazards and the accident producing processes. This approach is referred to as *analytical control by design and plans.* Methods used to support this strategy are future orientated, i.e. risk management measures like Probabilistic Safety Analysis (PSA), Probabilistic Risk Analysis (PRA), Human Reliability Analysis (HRA)

A combined *feedforward and feedback strategy* is used for concentrated sources of high hazards with slow change, aiming to control safety by an ongoing adjustment of feedforward methods according to experience gained by the use of feedback methods, the so called *control by evolutionary choice.*

A separate, though comparable, categorisation is introduced by Reason (1995) who distinguishes three different models of safety management according to their principal focus:

The *person model* is the traditional occupational safety approach focusing mainly on errors, unsafe acts and personal injuries. The underlying idea is that people are free to choose between safe or unsafe behaviour. Errors are attributed mainly to psychological factors such as inattention, poor motivation or lack of skills. Individuals are therefore the targets for safety management interventions.

The *engineering model* originates from traditional ergonomics, cognitive engineering and risk management. It is based on the idea that safety can be 'engineered' into systems reliability, since failures are seen as originating from man-machine mismatches. The model focuses on man-machine-interaction, i.e. the performance of operators and the safety related influence of the workplace. Safety is measured mainly by probabilistic risk and safety analysis methods.

The *organisational model* is linked to crisis management and can be considered as an extension of the engineering model. The underlying idea is that safety can be reached by the absence of latent factors which would increase the probability of human errors. Safety is measured by pro-active methods, like TRIPOD (Reason, 1995) and means a continuous control and adjustment of the system's basic processes, similar to the notion of Total Quality Management.

A comparison of Reason's and Rasmussen's categorisation for safety management approaches leads to the following conclusions: 'Empirical control by objective and the 'person model' are both within the traditional field of occupational safety. With the strategy of 'analytical control by design and plans' and the 'engineering model' the perspective is changed to high hazard industries, but still mainly on system functions and man-machine-interaction, leaving out organisational weaknesses. Approaches concentrating on latent factors can be considered under the 'organisational model' where the necessary control strategy is 'control by evolutionary choice', combining feedforward and feedback strategies.

Reason (1995) argues that a concentration on the 'person model' would probably result in an increase of organisational accidents with damage to the organisation and its environment, because measures are mainly directed to the operators in the 'sharp end' of production and might therefore lead to shortcuts in behaviour, thus endangering the system safety. This is a position which is supported by several other safety researchers claiming that the 'person model' is still the most influential one in accident analyses (Shealy, 1979; Benner, 1981 a and b; Hendrick and Benner, 1987). (For a discussion of these issues in a medical context, see Bogner, Chapter 5, and Taylor-Adams and Vincent, Chapter 6.)

Safety management with a feedforward strategy means assessing the risks of a system, foreseeing possible accidents and identifying possible weaknesses in order to improve the system defences by countermeasures. Usually quantitative methods are used here, but recently more qualitative approaches have gained ground, in an effort to introduce management and cultural aspects as well (Kirwan, 1998). In addition, there are methods for modelling technology (e.g., PSA), human contributions, (e.g., HRA) and some attempts to integrate both. An excellent overview and evaluation of different HRA techniques is presented by Kirwan (1996, 1997 a, b, c and d) and Kirwan *et al.* (1997). Safety management based on feedback strategies is conducted by gathering experience from operating, mainly through the analysis of accidents, incidents and near-misses (van der Schaaf, 1992). There are still only a few systematic accident analysis approaches and these are often contradicted by implicit theories of the investigators, which are often related to the person model (see below).

Safety management, through a combination of feedforward and feedback methods, can be seen as the implementation of an organisational learning system aiming to create and support a collective learning process. Carroll (in press) distinguishes in his model of organisational learning questions like what is learned, who does learn and how learning is based on a concept of learning as a generic feedback cycle (Draft and Weick, 1984; Schein, 1987; Argyris and Schon, 1996). The main elements of an organisational learning system are systematic tools for event analysis and reporting (Wilpert *et al.*, 1997). Thus, an organisational memory could be developed which assists members of the organisation and which influences future performance directly and indirectly by updating feedforward measures.

Inter-Organisational Concepts

Comprehensive safety management needs theories and concepts which link the environment and the focal organisation to each other, in order to understand their respective impact on system safety. In-depth analyses of several major industrial accidents showed that additional factors outside the focal organisation contributed to these accidents. The analysis of the capsising of the 'Herald of Free Enterprise' showed that, in addition to human errors, such as violations and managerial weaknesses, several extra-organisational contributing factors could be identified, for instance, 'harbour-management' 'ship-construction' and 'under-regulation'. Viewing safety in an exclusively organisational perspective remains therefore too narrow. An inter-organisational approach is needed which takes into account the interdependence of all the actors which contribute significantly to the system's outcome: 'its safety'.

The way that inter-organisational interdependence and problems of coordination and integration are related to safety of high hazard technologies has been demonstrated by so called network studies. For example, Wilpert and Fahlbruch (1998) carried out an intervention study aiming to introduce a 'Safety through Organizational Learning –SOL' approach in the German nuclear industry. The authors found that the main actors in the field were regulatory bodies (federal and state agencies), nuclear power plants belonging to different utilities, private consultant companies and the unions of employees in utilities. These actors are linked to each other in complex patterns of voluntary associations inhabiting structurally equivalent, i.e. similar positions in the network structure (DiMaggio and Powell, 1983), and also connected to each other in vertical and hierarchical patterns of relationships. This setting, the German Nuclear Safety System (GNSS), constitutes an inter-organisational field comprising a number of different individuals, organisations and regulatory bodies. The participants differ in size, goals, responsibility for safety, hierarchy and power with a wide range of mechanisms linking and coordinating the constituents of the field (Wilpert *et al.*, 1999).

The study of safety using traditional organisational concepts therefore needs to be complemented by theories and methods dealing with inter-organisational relationships. Concepts and methods of studying leadership, communication, centralisation, diagnosis and planned change for a higher level are needed to describe and explain the performance of inter-organisational relationships, as well as relationships within organisations. Observable trends of outsourcing of safety units (e.g. former British Rail and chemical and oil companies) lead to serious problems of responsibility, liability and safety management. As Baram (1998) has shown, the following types of change can have an enormous influence on system safety: down-sizing, out-sourcing, strategic alliances and deconstruction. Furthermore, in the view of new arising fields like genetic engineering or globalisation and internationalisation of markets, the primordial task will be to identify which actors belong to the whole system and how it functions before questions like liability and safety management can be discussed.

THEORETICAL UNDERPINNINGS: ACCIDENT GENESIS THEORIES

In which direction can we fruitfully direct our attention in the hope of finding some promising grounds to theoretically integrate the emerging field of system safety within industrial and organisational psychology? Fahlbruch and Wilpert (1999) discuss three promising theoretical perspectives: systems theory and cybernetics, the limits of information accessibility (Moray, in press) and theory of accident genesis. Here we limit ourselves to the third perspective as having the most immediate relevance to medicine. The actual application of accident analysis is discussed elsewhere in this book (see Bogner, Chaper 5 and Taylor-Adams and Vincent, Chapter 6).

Accident Genesis Theories

The reaction to and the treatment of accidents is mainly determined by the underlying accident causation theories and assumptions. They lay down, either explicitly or implicitly, the limits of accident investigation, i.e., which data are gathered and which are skipped, what kind of analysis is performed, or whether a search for one single root cause is carried out or a search for many contributing factors. Furthermore, the theory influences which 'causes' are reported and which recommendations are proposed and therefore which quality of learning from experience and which enhancement of system safety can be achieved.

Since the beginning of this century a number of accident causation theories have been developed, mainly dealing with occupational accidents (for reviews see Hale and Hale, 1972; Benner, 1975; Smillie and Ayoub, 1976). Nearly all of these theories originate from the field of occupational safety and focus on the individual and their errors or unsafe acts. Two conceptualisations are of particular importance to current theorising. First, the event-based model by Benner (1995) defines an accident as "not a single event, but rather a transformation process by which a homeostatic activity is interrupted with accompanying unintentional harm.

The critical point is that an accident is a process involving interacting elements and certain necessary or sufficient conditions". Secondly, the energy flow model (Johnson, 1973) emphasises elements such as energy, barriers and targets rather than the process and postulates that accidents are defined as an unwanted transfer of energy producing unwanted losses (injuries, damages or degradation of ongoing processes). Accidents occur because of inadequate or missing barriers / controls. In an evaluation of accident models and investigation methodologies, these two models were rated best by Benner (1975) according to ten dimensions, such as being realistic, definitive, satisfying, comprehensive, consistent and functional.

Approaches to accident investigation can be described from various perspectives: whether the accident is viewed as a single event or a chain of events (Benner, 1981 a and b) or according to their degree of standardisation (Shealy, 1979; Fahlbruch and Wilpert, 1997). Other criteria for the evaluation of accident analysis methods are their approach to overcoming shortcuts and biases in the human search for causal relationships (Fahlbruch and Wilpert, 1997; Reason, 1995; Carroll, in press) or their underlying theoretical approach (Becker *et al.*, 1996), which determines the stop rule for the investigation (Rasmussen, 1991b). Reviews of accident analysis methods can be found in Ferry (1988), and Becker *et al.* (1996). Since accidents are relatively infrequent events, recently safety research and safety management is extended to the analysis of near-accidents and near-misses (van der Schaaf, 1992, 1996 a and b, 1997; van Vuuren *et al.*, 1997). The analysis of events with less negative consequences leads also to a desirable shift from the search for scapegoats or someone to blame towards the identification of underlying contributing factors (Wilpert *et al.*, 1997).

Reason (1990a) extended accident causation theory to several levels within the organisation. He assumes that in high-hazard organisations, defence-in-depth-systems preclude the possibility that one unsafe act by an operator can cause a systems breakdown: additional weaknesses in the organisation are necessary for the occurrence of accidents. Reason (1990b) introduces the concept of active and latent failure. Active failures are associated with the 'front-line' operators and lead to immediate adverse effects, constituting a trigger function, whereas latent failures are associated with persons who are not involved in 'front-line' activities, e.g. decision makers, whose erroneous action could be unrecognised for a long time period, weakening the system functions like resident pathogens. He concludes that fallible decisions by top level management, deficiencies by line management, psychological precursors of unsafe acts, unsafe acts of operators as well as inadequate system defences together create a limited window for an accident occurrence path. This conceptualisation leads to an extended scope of perspective which takes explicitly into account the management contribution and therefore can be categorised as an organisational model.

A partial extension of Reason's model through an addition of environmental contribution is postulated by a German research group (Wilpert *et al.*, 1994; Becker *et al.*, 1996; Wilpert *et al.*, 1997). Coming from the socio-technical system approach, the research group defines five different subsystems in the nuclear industry: individual, team, organisation/management, extra-organisational environment and technology. Each of these subsystems and their interaction are seen to influence safety. In line with Reason's accident causation theory (1990a) it is postulated that accidents occur because of the interaction of directly and indirectly contributing factors. Directly contributing factors trigger the event, whereas indirectly contributing factors promote the occurrence and virulence of directly contributing factors and weaken the system. Contributing factors can originate from each of the subsystems and their interactions. Two points are of particular importance: first, the renouncement of the term 'error' or 'failure'. This is done for several reasons: the term indicates liability or blame, an 'error' can be defined only according to consequences and identified therefore only by hind-sight. This leads to difficulties with regard to 'failures' such as erroneous management decisions taken years ago. Second, with the explicit expansion to extra-organisational factors, an attempt is made to facilitate the explanation of accident occurrences from an inter-organisational perspective.

A major problem of accident analysis methods is their lack of proper evaluation. Once a method is developed it is usually assessed in terms of its usability and then applied to the analysis of real-life events. There is a clear danger of obtaining arbitrary results. The analysis of an accident is always a retrospective social reconstruction process, starting with insufficient information about what happened and resulting in inferences about the causes / contributing factors. Traditional validity measures cannot easily be applied to this process. Therefore, Wilpert *et al.* (1997) introduced a stepwise evaluation of their accident analysis approach SOL. They used experts' judgements and experimental studies, as well as near-miss re-analyses to show that using SOL trained practitioners are able to identify directly and indirectly contributing factors

In summary, starting from an individual and technical perspective, the scope is widened to the organisational influence, with little attention yet paid to inter-organisational influences. The majority of accident analyses is still conducted on the basis of often implicit underlying person or technology oriented models. Accident causation theories are still vague as regards the exact nature of organisational or inter-organisational dysfunction. There is a need for theories that model the overall day to day functioning of organisations and an even greater need for the modelling of inter-organisational relationships to explain deviations which can lead to system breakdowns.

CONCLUSIONS AND APPLICATIONS FOR MEDICINE

This overview of the literature on system safety illustrates its basic inter-disciplinary nature. Our starting point was to outline the difference between occupational and system safety, the former dealing with intra-organisational incidents and accidents while the latter considers the interrelationship between organisational and extra-organisational factors. This new focus was attributed to the emergence of accelerating technologies in large scale socio-technical systems with high hazard potential. Safety science can be described in five different research strands: a pessimistic and optimistic views of safety control, a holistic consideration of safety as a characteristic of organisational culture, safety as a consequence of managerial strategies and techniques and system safety as a result of properly functioning inter-organisational relationships. These five traditions are not mutually exclusive but overlap and influence each other.

It would be premature and foolhardy to say which of these paradigms may be most fruitful in healthcare, but some preliminary remarks may be helpful. Perrow's identification of systems with particularly high hazard potential may certainly be of relevance in medicine, particularly in technologically sophisticated acute medicine, though the solution of simply not using such technologies is unlikely to be feasible in healthcare. The model high reliability organisations may certainly be useful in identifying potentially important personal and organisational factors which may be correlated with safe or unsafe clinical care, or with other measures of quality. The idea of safety culture is almost completely unexplored within healthcare, beyond the assumption that most clinicians have the interests of their patients are heart. The development of a clinical equivalent of a questionnaire to measure safety culture would be of considerable interest and could later be linked to other measures of quality of care, both process and outcome. Safety management *per se* is little discussed, though there are of course a large number of methods and approaches in healthcare that aim to enhance quality and, by implication, safety. There is, however, little explicit discussion of fundamental approaches to safety, such as those of Rasmussen or Hale and few attempts to draw on the general safety literature.

Harm to patients and adverse outcomes of all kinds have always been of concern to clinicians, but are now acquiring a much higher public profile. In Britain, Germany and elsewhere there is now a much greater willingness to study and reflect on the role of human error in healthcare and the causes of adverse events and, in parallel, a growing acknowledgement of the importance of risk management in a clinical context. Risk management in Britain and most other European countries is still at an early stage of development, with little attention given to research and less still to theory. However, Reason's model of organisational accidents has certainly been influential (Leape, 1994; Vincent *et al.*, 1998) and interest in the safety problems of other domains in growing. Risk management in healthcare may provide the most fruitful point of contact for human factors and safety researchers and practitioners. The challenge for them is to understand the particular perspective and culture of healthcare. Conversely, clinicians and healthcare researchers face quite a challenge in attempting to understand the material reviewed in this chapter. This chapter, and indeed this book, suggest that both sides will benefit by collaboration and exploration of each other's areas.

REFERENCES

ACSNI Study Group on Human Factors. (1993). *Organising for Safety* (THIRD Report to Health and Safety Commission. ACSNI Study Group on Human Factors, Advisory Committee on the Safety of Nuclear Installations). Health and Safety Commission, London.

Argyris, C., and D. Schon (1996). *Organizational Learning II; Theory, Method, and Practice.* Addison-Wesley, Reading, MA.

Baram, M. (1998). Process safety management and the implications of organizational change. In: A. Hale and M. Baram (eds.), *Safety Management and the Challenge of Organisational Change.* Elsevier, Amsterdam.

Becker, G., S. Hoffmann, B. Wilpert, R. Miller, B. Fahlbruch, M. Fank, M. Freitag, H.-G. Giesa, and L. Schleifer (1996). *Analyse der Ursachen von "menschlichem Fehlverhalten" beim Betrieb von Kernkraftwerken.* Der Bundesminister für Umwelt, Naturschutz und Reaktorsicherheit, Bonn, BMU-1996-454.

Benner, L. (1975). Accident theory and accident investigation. In: *Proceedings of the Annual Seminar*, pp. 148-154. Society of Air Safety Investigators, Ottawa.

Benner, L. (1981a). Accident perceptions: Their implications for accident investigators. *isasi forum*, spring, 13-17.

Benner, L. (1981b). Methodological biases which undermine accident investigations. *Proceedings of International Society of Air Safety Investigators International Symposium*, 1-5.

Benner, L. (1985). Rating accident models and investigation methodologies. *Journal of Safety Research*, **16**, 105-126.

Brascamp, M. H., L. J. B. Koehorst and J. F. J. van Steen (1993). Management factors in safety. In: *Safety and Reliability Assessment - an Integral Approach* (P. Kafke and J. Wolf, eds.), pp. 35-48. Elsevier, Amsterdam,

Büttner, T. (1997). *Erheben von Sicherheitskultur. Darstellung und Analyse gebräuchlicher Verfahren und Instrumente.* Technische Universität Berlin, Diplomarbeit.

Carroll, J. S. (in press). Incident reviews in high-hazard industries: Sensemaking and learning under ambiguity and accountability. *Industrial and Environmental Crisis Quarterly.*

Cox, S. and T. Cox (1991). The structure of employee attitudes to safety: A European example. *Work and Stress*, **5**, 93-106.

DiMaggio, P. J., and W. W. Powell (1983). The iron cage revisited: Institutional isomorphism and collective rationality in organizational fields. *American Sociological Review*, **48**, 147-160.

Draft, R. L. and K. E. Weick (1984). Toward a model of organizations as interpretation system. *Academy of Management Review*, **9**, 284-295.

Fahlbruch, B. and B.Wilpert (1997). Event Analysis as Problem Solving Process. In: *After the Event - From Accident Analysis to Organisational Learning* (A. Hale, M. Freitag and B. Wilpert, eds.), pp. 113-130. Elsevier, Amsterdam.

Fahlbruch, B. and B. Wilpert, (1999). System safety – an emerging field for I/O psychology. In: *International Review of Industrial and Organizational Psychology (Vol.14)* (L. Cooper and I.T. Robertson, eds.), pp. 55-93. Wiley, Chichester.

Ferry, T. S. (1988). *Modern Accident Investigation and Analysis.* Wiley, Chichester.

Freud, S. (1914). *Psychopathology of Everyday Life*, Ernest Ben, London.

Groeneweg, J. (1992). *Controlling the Controllable. The Management of Safety.* DSWO Press, Leiden. 150-159.

Haber, S. B., D. S. Metlay and D. A. Crouch (1990). Influence of Organizational Factors on Safety. *Proceedings of the Human Factors Society*, 871-875.

Hale, A. R. (1985). *The Human Paradox in Technology and Safety. Inaugural Lecture.* Safety Science Group, Delft University of Technology.

Hale, A. R. and M. Hale (1972). *A Review of the Industrial Accident Research Literature.* HMSO, London.

Hale, A. R., B. H. J. Heming, J. Carthey and B. Kirwan (1997). Modelling of safety management systems. *Safety Science*, **26**, 121-140.

Heimann, C. F. L. (1993). Understanding the Challenger disaster: Organizational structure and the design of reliable systems. *American Political Science Review*, **87**, 421-438.

Hendrick, K. and L. Benner (1987). *Investigating Accidents with STEP.* Dekker, New York.

Hovden, J. (1996). Internal control of safety, health and environment (SHE) in industry: An effective alternative to direct regulation and control by authorities? In: *Probabilistic Safety Assessment and Management'96* (C. Cacciabue and A. Papazoglou, eds.), pp. 683-689 Springer, London.

Hovden, J. and R. K. Tinmannisvik (1990). Internal control: A strategy for occupational safety and health. Experiences from Norway. *Journal of Occupational Accidents*, **12**, 21-30.

Hoyos, C. Graf and F. Ruppert (1993). *Der Fragebogen zur Sicherheitsdiagnose (FSD) - Entwicklung und Erprobung eines verhaltensorientierten Verfahrens für die betriebliche Sicherheitsarbeit.* Huber, Bern.

INSAG. (1991). *Safety Culture.* International Atomic Energy Agency, Vienna.

Johnson, W. (1973). *The Management Oversight and Risk Tree -MORT* ((SAN 821-2)). US Atomic Energy Commission, Germantown, MD.

Kirwan, B. (1996). The Validation of three human reliability quantification techniques - THERP, HEART and JHEDI: Part 1 - Technique descriptions and validation issues. *Applied Ergonomics*, **27**, 359-373.

Kirwan, B. (1997a). The development of a nuclear chemical plant human reliability management approach: HRMS and JHEDI. *Reliability Engineering and System Safety*, **56**, 107-133.

Kirwan, B. (1997b). The validation of three human reliability quantification techniques - THERP, HEART and JHEDI: Practical aspects of the usage of the techniques. *Applied Ergonomics*, **28**, 27-39.

Kirwan, B. (1997c). Validation of human reliability assessment techniques: Part 2 - Validation results. *Safety Science*, **27**, 43-75.

Kirwan, B. (1997d). Validation of human reliability assessment techniques: Part 1 - Validation issues. *Safety Science*, **27**, 25-41.

Kirwan, B. (1998). Safety management assessment and task analysis: A missing link? In: *Safety Management and the Challenge of Organisational Change* (A. Hale and M. Baram, eds.). Elsevier, Amsterdam.

Kjellén, U. (1982). Evaluation of safety information systems in six medium-sized and large firms. *Journal of Occupational Accidents*, **3**, 273-288.

La Porte, T. R. (1994). Large technical systems, institutional surprises, and challenges to political legitimacy. *Technology in Society*, **16**, 269-288.

La Porte, T. R., and D. S. Metlay (1996). Hazards and institutional trustworthiness: Facing a deficit of trust. *Public Administration Review*, **56**, 341-347.

Leape L L. (1994). Error in medicine. *Journal of the American Medical Association*, **272**(23), 1851-1857.

Maxwell R. (1984). Quality assessment in health. *British Medical Journal*, **288**, 1470-1472.

Mitroff, I. I., T. Pauchant, M. Finney and C. Pearson (1989). Do (some) organizations cause their own crises? The cultural profiles of crisis-prone vs crisis-prepared organizations. *Industrial Crisis Quarterly*, **3**(4), 269-283.

Moray, N. (in press). Is the future like the past and can we reach it from here? In: *Coping with Accelerating Socio-Technical Systems* (B. Kirwan, L. Norros and B. Fahlbruch, eds.). Elsevier, Amsterdam.

Nichols, M. and A. Marcus (1990). *Empirical Studies of Candidate Leading Indicators of Safety in Nuclear Power Plants: An Expanded View of Human Factors Research*. Paper presented at the 34th Annual Meeting, Proceedings of the Human Factors Society.

Norman, D. A. (1981). Categorization of action slips. *Psychological Review*, **88**(1), 1-15.

Ostrom, L., C. Wilhelmsen and B. Kaplan (1993). Assessing Safety Culture. *Nuclear Safety*, **34**(2), 163-172.

Perrow, C. (1984). *Normal Accidents: Living with High-Risk Technologies*. Basic Books, New York.

Rasmussen, J. (1987). Cognitive control and human error mechanisms. In: *New Technologies and Human Error* (J. Rasmussen, K. Duncan, and J. Leplat, eds.), pp. 53-61. Wiley, Chichester.

Rasmussen, J. (1991a). *Safety Control: Some Basic Distinctions and Research Issues in High Hazard Low Risk Operation*. Paper presented at the NeTWork workshop on Risk Management, Bad Homburg, May 1991.

Rasmussen, J. (1991b). Event analysis and the problem of causality. In: *Distributed Decision Making: Cognitive Models for Cooperative Work* (J. Rasmussen, B. Brehmer and J. Leplat, eds.), pp. 251-259. Wiley, Chichester,.

Reason, J. (1990a). *Human Error*. Cambridge University Press, Cambridge.

Reason, J. (1990b). The contribution of latent human failures to the breakdown of complex systems. *Philosophical Transactions of the Royal Society London*, **327**, 475-484.

Reason, J. T. (1995). Understanding adverse events: human factors. In: *Clinical risk management* (C. A. Vincent, ed.), pp. 31-54. BMJ Publications, London:.

Reason, J. (in press). Managing the Risks of Organizational Accidents. Ashgate, Aldenshot.

Roberts, K. H. (1990). Some characteristics of one type of high reliability organization. *Organization Science*, **1**(2), 160-176.

Roberts, K. H. (1992). Structuring to facilitate migrating decisions in reliability enhancing organizations. *Top Management and Executive Leadership in High Technology. Advances in Global High-Technology Management*, **2**, 171-191.

Roberts, K. H., S. K. Stout and J. J. Halpern (1994). Decision dynamics in two high reliability military organizations. *Management Science*, **40**(5), 614-624.

Rochlin, G. I. (1989). Informal organizational networking as a crisis-avoidance strategy: US naval flight operations as a case study. *Industrial Crisis Quarterly*, **3**, 159-176.

Rochlin, G. I. (1993). Defining "high reliability" organizations in practice: A taxonomic prologue. In: *New Challenges to Understanding Organizations* (K. H. Roberts, ed.), pp. 11-31. Macmillan, New York,

Roland, H. E., and B. Moriarty (1990). *System Safety Engineering and Management*. Wiley, New York.

Sackmann, S. (1983). Organisationskultur: Die unsichtbare Einflußgröße. *Gruppendynamik*, **14**, 393-406.

Sagan, S. D. (1993). *The Limits of Safety. Organizations, Accidents, and Nuclear Weapons*. Princeton University Press, Princeton, NJ.

Schein, E. H. (1985). *Organizational Culture and Leadership*. Jossey-Bass, San Francisco.

Schein, E. H. (1987). *Process Consultation, Vol. II: Lessons for Managers and Consultants*. Addison-Wesley, Reading, MA.

Shealy, J. E. (1979). Impact of theory of accident causation on intervention strategies. *Proceedings of the Human Factors Society*, 23rd Annual Meeting, 225-229.

Sheehy, N. P. and A. J. Chapman (1987). Industrial accidents. In: *International Review of Industrial and Organizational Psychology* (C. L. Cooper and I. T. Robertson eds.), pp. 201-227. Wiley, Chichester,.

Shrivastava, P. (1987). *Bhopal: Anatomy of a Crisis*. Ballinger, Cambridge.

Slovic, P. (1993). Perceived risk, trust, and democracy. *Risk Analysis*, **13**(6), 675-682.

Smillie, R. J. and Ayoub, M. A. (1976). Accident causation theories: A simulation approach. *Journal of Occupational Accidents*, **1**, 47-68.

Starbuck, W. H. and F. J. Milliken (1988). Challenger: Fine-tuning the odds until something breaks. *Journal of Management Studies*, **25**(4), 319-340.

Taylor D. (1996). Quality and professionalism in health care; a review of current initiatives in the NHS. *British Medical Journal*, **312**, 626-629.

Turner, B. A. (1978). *Man-Made Disasters*. Wykeham, London.

van der Schaaf, T. W. (1992). *Near Miss Reporting in the Chemical Process Industry*. (Dissertation), Eindhoven.

van der Schaaf, T. W. (1996a). Human recovery of errors in man-machine systems. *Proccedings of the International Conference and Workshop on Process Safety Management and Inherently Safer Processes*. Center for Chemical Process Safety of American Institute of Chemical Engineers, New York, 356-365.

van der Schaaf, T. W. (1996b). PRISMA: A risk management tool based on incident analysis. *Proccedings of the International Conference and Workshop on Process Safety Management and Inherently Safer Processes*. Center for Chemical Process Safety of the American Intitute of Chemical Engineers, New York, 242-251.

van der Schaaf, T. W. (1997). Human error and system safety: Can lessons from process control be applied to other domains? In: *Proceedings of the CSAPC*, (S. Bagnara, E. Hollnagel, M. Mariani, and L. Norros, eds.), pp. 66-70. CNR, Rome.

van Vuuren, W., C. E. Shea and T. W. van der Schaaf (1997). *The Development of an Incident Analysis Tool for the Medical Field* (Report EUT/BDK/85). Eindhoven University of Technology, Eindhoven.

Vaughan, D. (1996). *The Challenger Launch Decision: Risky Technology, Culture, and Deviance at NASA*. Chicago University Press, Chicago.

Vincent, C.A. (1997). Risk, safety and the dark side of quality. *British Medical Journal*, **314**, 1775-6.

Vincent, C. A., S. Taylor-Adams and N. Stanhope (1998). A framework for the analysis of risk and safety in medicine. *British Medical Journal*, **316**, 1154-1157.

von Bertalannfy, L. (1950). The theory of open systems in physics and biology. *Science*, **3**, 23-29.

Weimer, H. (1922). Wesen und Arten der Fehler (I. Teil). *Zeitschrift für pädagogische Psychologie*, **24**, 17-25.

Wilpert, B. (1991). *System Safety and Safety Culture*, Paper presented at the joint IAEA, IIASA meeting on "The Influence of Organization and Management on the Safety of NPPs and Other Industrial Systems", 18 -20 March 1991, Vienna, Austria.

Wilpert, B., G. Becker, H. Maimer, R. Miller, B. Fahlbruch, R. Baggen, A. Gans, I. Leiber and S. Szameitat (1997). *Umsetzung und Erprobung von Vorschlägen zur Einbeziehung von Human Factors (HF) bei der Meldung und Ursachenanalyse in Kernkraftwerken.* Endbericht SR 2039/8, Bundesamt für Strahlenschutz, Salzgitter.

Wilpert, B. and B. Fahlbruch (1998). Safety related interventions in interorganisational fields. In: *Safety Management and the Challenge of Organisational Change* (A. Hale and M. Baram, eds.). Elsevier, Amsterdam.

Wilpert, B., B. Fahlbruch, R. Miller, R. Baggen and A. Gans (1999). Interorganizational development in the German nuclear safety system. In: *Nuclear Safety: A Human Factors Perspective* (J. Misumi, B. Wilpert and R. Miller, eds.). Taylor and Francis, London.

Wilpert, B., M. Fank, B. Fahlbruch, M. Freitag, H.-G. Giesa, R. Miller, and G. Becker (1994). *Weiterentwicklung der Erfassung und Auswertung von meldepflichtigen Vorkommnissen und sonstigen registrierten Ereignissen beim Betrieb von Kernkraftwerken hinsichtlich menschlichen Fehlverhaltens.* Bundesminister für Umwelt, Naturschutz und Reaktorsicherheit, BMU-1996-457, Bonn.

Wilpert, B., and P. Klumb (1991). Störfall in Biblis A. *Zeitschrift für Arbeitswissenschaft*, **45**, 51-54.

Zimolong, B. (1996). Ganzheitliches Sicherheitsmanagement im bergmännischen Tagebau. In: *Psychologie der Arbeitssicherhei* (B. Ludborzs, H. Nold and B. Rüttinger, eds.), pp. 610-611. Asanger, Heidelberg.

ACKNOWLEDGEMENT

This chapter is based on an earlier chapter by Babette Fahlbruch and Bernhard Wilpert, 'System safety – an emerging field for I/O psychology'. In C.L. Cooper, and I.T. Robertson (Eds.), International Review of Industrial and Organizational Psychology (1999).

CHAPTER 2

THE CONCEPT OF HUMAN ERROR: IS IT USEFUL FOR THE DESIGN OF SAFE SYSTEMS IN HEALTHCARE?

Jens Rasmussen,HURECON, Denmark

INTRODUCTION

Analyses of accidents have often concluded that 'human error' is a determining factor in 70-80% of the cases. Furthermore, multiple contributing errors and faults are normally found because several defences against accident have been used to protect a hazardous process. Typically, it is also concluded that the 'root cause' of the accident was a human error on the part of a person involved directly in the dynamic flow of events, a pilot, a process operator or a train driver.

Consequently, a great deal of effort has been spent on improving safety by enhancing training schemes, introducing safety campaigns motivating the work force to be safety conscious and improving work system design so as to prevent repetitions of the human errors identified from analysis of past incidents and accidents. In addition, considerable resources have been spent on research into human error and comprehensive programmes have been established to define and categorise human behaviour in terms of errors, without any significant success. Reliable 'human error' data bases still do not exist and bench mark exercises to validate human reliability prediction have shown orders of magnitude variation in estimates due to unreliable behavioural models (Amendola, 1989).

Analyses of several large-scale accidents, such as Flixborough, Zeebrügge, Clapham Junction and Chernobyl, have shown show that such accidents cannot be explained by a stochastic coincidence of independent events. Accidents are more likely to be caused by a systematic migration toward accident by a company operating in an aggressive, competitive environment or an organisation working under time and funding pressure (Rasmussen, 1993a, 94). During such periods, success depends on an exploitation of the benefits accruing from operating at the fringes of the usual, accepted practice. Closing in on the boundaries of established practice and exploring the benefits of working under time constraints or during financial crises necessarily implies a risk of crossing the limits of safe practice. Similar conditions are also likely to be found within health care systems during periods of political pressure toward cost-effectiveness.

Design of safer systems, in healthcare and in general, may be enhanced if we reconsider the concept of human error and analyse in depth the mechanisms that shape organisational response to the pressures of a dynamic, competitive society.

ERRORS AND EXPERTISE

Actually, the concept of 'human error' turns out to be very elusive. On closer study, the frequent allocation of accidental causes to human error appears to be subjective and guided by the tool box of the analyst. This is a simple reflection of the nature of causal analysis and the fact that no objective stop rule exists to terminate the causal back tracking in search of a root cause. The search stops when an event is found for which a cure is known to the analyst (Rasmussen, 1990a,b), and you can always blame the actors involved in the dynamic course of events.

Behaviour patterns classified after the fact as 'errors', tend, instead, to be an indication of actors exploring the boundaries of acceptable performance in an unkind environment. This perception of errors as being a reflection of efforts to learn to interact effectively with an environment has long roots. Already Ernest Mach (1905, p. 84) notes:

"Knowledge and error flow from the same mental sources, only success can tell the one from the other."

Selz (1922) also found that errors in problem solving were not stochastic events, but had to be seen as being the results of solution trials. An important implication of this is that experts on the run typically make more errors than novices cautiously seeking the tricks of the trade. Hadamard, the French mathematician, states (1945, p. 49):

"-- in our domain, we do not have to ponder with errors. Good mathematicians, when they make them, which is not infrequent, soon perceive and correct them. As for me (and mine is the case of many mathematicians), I make many more of them than my students do; only I always correct them so that no trace of them remains in the final result. The reason for that is that whenever an error has been made, insight - that same scientific sensibility we have spoken of - warns me that my calculations do not look as they ought to".

Rather than studying errors we ought to focus on strategies to recover from unsuccessful explorations. The interaction of experts with a work environment involves several different cognitive levels of control (Rasmussen, 1983) that are organised in a three level hierarchy. The lowest level is the *skill-based level,* taking care of work routines that run without conscious control. At the next level, the *rule-based level,* control depends on know-how. This means a sequence of automated routines are organised according to a rule or plan known to be operational from previous occasions. When no plan or rule is available, behavioural control moves to the *knowledge-based level* and a plan must be generated, based on basic understanding of the relational properties of the work system that makes it possible to predict the results of intended actions. The evolution of expertise manifests itself in the distribution of error mechanisms at all levels of the cognitive control of performance.

For problem solving at the *knowledge-based level,* planning depends on prediction and an opportunity for testing hypotheses is important for the development of expertise. It is typically expected that qualified personnel such as process operators and surgeons can and will test their diagnostic hypotheses conceptually before acting because the effects of their actions may be irreversible and hazardous. This may, however, be an unrealistic assumption. No explicit, objective stop rule exists to guide the termination of conceptual analysis and the start of action. This means that the definition of errors, as seen from the perspective of a problem solver, is very arbitrary. Actions which are quite rational and important during the search for information and the test of a hypothesis may appear to be unacceptable mistakes in hindsight, without access to the details of the situation.

This situation is often found when analysing cases of medical 'accidents'. Diagnosis and treatment of patients can be compared to piloting patients through troubled water (Paget, 1988). The state of health of patients depends on numerous obscure conditions and treatment may have many side effects which are difficult, if not impossible, to predict. A diagnosis, therefore, has the character of a hypothesis and treatment that of a hypothesis test. Frequently, the knowledge needed for a proper diagnosis is present too late and it is only after the fact that a stop rule to guide the termination of data collection prior to action becomes evident. The question is: when to stop thinking and start action? The answer depends on a trade-off between indecisiveness and the risk of a premature decision, a trade-off that depends on many subtle situational factors that usually cannot be made explicit at a later point in time.

The difficulty of defining errors in problem solving scenarios becomes evident when considering erroneous decisions in scientific research. Consequently, erroneous scientific decisions have been studied under the label of 'anomalies' (Star *et al.*, 1986). The question is, under what conditions is a scientific concept or hypothesis useful and when does it become obsolete and erroneous? This question is highlighted by the frequent shift in recommendations for healthy diets depending on the latest MD thesis.

Also for *rule-based control* of activities during familiar work situations for which accepted procedures exist, there will be ample opportunities for modification of such procedures. The development of expert know-how and rules-of-thumb depends on adaptation governed by an empirical correlation of convenient cues with successful acts. During normal familiar work, actors are immersed in the context for long periods, they know the flow of activity and the useful action alternatives by heart. Therefore they need not consult the complete set of defining attributes before acting in a familiar situation. Instead, guided by the path of least resistance, they will seek no more information than is necessary for discrimination among the perceived alternatives for action in the particular situation. Thus, when situations change, for instance due to disturbances or faults in the system, reliance on the usual cues which are no longer valid may lead to error. Again, a trade-off takes place: speed versus the risk of a latent change of context that may make the actor's know-how obsolete.

In this way, information collection for a familiar diagnostic task will be guided by the perceived repertoire of relevant actions. Therefore, diagnostic observations made by a medical doctor during one phase of a patient's treatment will be unreliable for colleagues having different roles and action alternatives. When doctors have different roles and tool boxes it follows that they also have different biases during their information search (Rasmussen, 1993b; Rasmussen and Pedersen, 1991).

Even for highly automated, subconscious work routines at the *skill-based level*, evolution of behavioural patterns will take place according to a subconscious exploration of the properties of the environment. In a manual skill, fine-tuning depends upon continuous experiments to match the patterns of movement to the temporal and spatial features of the task environment. Behavioural optimisation is guided by criteria such as speed and smoothness and how far this adaptation can be accepted is only indicated by the once-in-a-while experience gained when crossing the tolerance limits, i.e. by the experience of slips. At this level, therefore, expertise depends on a speed-accuracy trade-off. Errors have a function in maintaining a skill at its proper level and they cannot be considered a separable category of events in a causal chain because they are integral parts of a feed-back loop.

An example is the monitoring task during anesthesia. A literature review by Rizzi (1990) showed that slack monitoring is claimed to be an important contributor to the complication rate during anesthesia. However, the impact of monitoring and monitoring devices did not seem to be validated through clinical trials or quality assurance procedures. Likewise, human adaptation to monitoring requirements had not been considered in the published accounts. The individual patient's need for monitoring varies within very wide limits. It will not be possible to extend the normal monitoring effort to cover all contingencies and the tail of the distribution will end up as being 'monitoring errors' after the fact. There is no other way to control the proper monitoring effort other than to watch the error rate. Work-load pressure will necessarily cause the staff to readjust their monitoring effort until the limit of acceptable performance is found, unless a way can be found to show the set of relevant attributes by an integrated visual pattern. We will return to this point below.

Considering that errors therefore reflect a necessary adaptive trade-off, the present efforts to apply general business management theories to healthcare systems in order to rationalise operation with a focus on cost effectiveness, raise the fundamental question whether accidents are only indicators of the limits of acceptable work pressure. In that case, safety research focusing on the operative level cannot remove accidents but will only serve to choose the context in which to expect their occurrence. What will happen when a new business manager reorganises a hospital for cost-effectiveness and lays-off a couple of hundred nurses? A recent critical review of the effects of this trend on public healthcare is found in Rees and Rodley (1995).

If the hypothesis is accepted that experts tend to minimise the number of action alternatives in order to eliminate the need for choice and decision during normal work and that errors are a necessary part of this adaptation, then the trick in the design of reliable systems is to counteract the fixation on stereotypic practice by making sure that the human actors maintain sufficient flexibility to cope with system aberrations, i.e., not to try to constrain their outlook by training 'proper procedures'. It appears to be essential that actors maintain 'contact' with hazards in such a way that they will be familiar with the boundary to loss of control and will learn to recover. That is also the basic message of Hadamard's statement.

When attempts are made to design 'safe' systems by making the margins between normal practice and loss of control as wide as possible, the odds are that the actors will not be able to sense the boundaries under normal circumstances and, very likely, that the new boundaries will be more abrupt and mistakes irreversible. When radar was introduced to increase safety at sea, the result was not increased safety but more efficient transportation under bad weather conditions. The introduction of anti-locking car brakes appeared not to decrease the accident rate but to affect driving speed and abruptness (Rasmussen, 1990b). A basic design question then is: how can reversible boundaries of acceptable performance be established that will give feedback to a learning mode, i.e., absorb violations in a mode of graceful degradation of the opportunities to recover.

The conclusion here is that we need field studies of the normal behaviour and analyses of the behaviour-shaping constraints and pressures found in specific work domains in order to understand migration toward the boundary of safe practice, together with efforts to identify the recovery strategies that experts use to develop the insight and sensibility that was mentioned by Hadamard. Recently, important progress has been made in this direction in the healthcare arena. Dominguez and colleagues have studied laparoscopic cholecystectomy with a focus on the decision when to convert to an open procedure if the anatomy cannot be clearly visualised through the video camera (Dominguez, 1998; Dominguez *et al.*, in press). They showed a recording of the visual field as it was available to the surgeon during an actual, critical case and asked 20 surgeons to consider the decision when to go to the open procedure. This decision is a difficult trade-off, depending on an explorative identification of the boundary of safe operation and the strategies for recovery available to the surgeon, relying heavily on the level of expertise. Their research represents an important attempt to study the exploration of boundary conditions and development of recovery strategies. The trend in this direction was also demonstrated at the 1998 US National Patient Safety Foundation workshop, concluding that studies of success stories are as important as failures (Cook *et al.*, 1998). It was also concluded that safety in healthcare is a social, organisational problem, and that research should not be focused on human error on the part of actors at the operative level.

THE ORGANISATIONAL ISSUE

The next issue to consider is the organisational response to pressure from a dynamic and competitive environment.

In most situations, staff have many possible ways to work efficiently. As they explore the work environment, guided by subjective process criteria such as cost effectiveness, work load, time spent, etc., they gain experience in maximising the efficiency of their work methods. Unfortunately, these aspects of the work process itself are immediately experienced while the ultimate outcome of the process can be considerably delayed, obscure and dependent on many other activities. Short-cuts and tricks-of-the-trade will frequently evolve and be very efficient under normal conditions, while they will be judged serious human errors when, under special circumstances, they lead to serious accidents.

The Clapham Junction railway accident (HMSO, 1989) presents a clear example of how a safe work procedure for signal system modifications, including multiple precautions against human errors, gradually degenerates due to adaptation to a locally more efficient work practice. In this case, for instance, safety checks following modifications of signal system wiring were planned to be independently performed by three different persons, the technician, his supervisor and the system engineer. Work force constraints and tight work schedules following a reorganisation, however, led to a more 'efficient' division of work. The supervisor took part in the actual, physical work and the independent check by him as well as by the engineer was abandoned. In addition, the technician integrated the check, i.e., a 'wire-count', into the modification task itself, although it was intended to be his final separate check. In short, adaptation to a more effective division of work under time pressure causes the redundancy required for high reliability to deteriorate.

Another illustrative case is the unfortunate capsizing of the ferry Herald of Free Enterprise at Zeebrügge (HMSO, 1987), see figure 2.1. In this case, an organisational pressure toward cost effectiveness in a highly competitive environment caused several decision makers to run risks. These cases illustrate how accidents are caused by the side effects of decisions made by different actors distributed in different organisations, at different levels of society and during activities at different points in time. These decision makers are deeply immersed in their normal, individual work context. Their daily activities are not functionally coupled, only an accident as observed after the fact connects their performance into a particular coupled pattern. By their various independent decisions and acts, they shape a causal path through the landscape along which an accidental course of events sooner or later may be released, very likely by a normal variation in somebody's work performance – which will then probably be judged the 'root cause' of the accident once it has occurred.

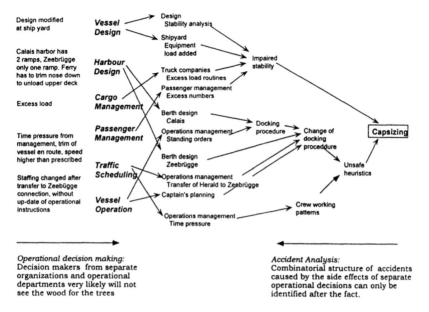

Figure 2.1. The capsizing of the ferry Herald of Free Enterprise at Zeebrügge, 1987, represents an example of the operation of an organisation under harsh competitive pressure.

The mechanisms illustrated by such examples now seem to be increasingly critical, since we are facing some changes of the general conditions of safety and risk management:

- Companies and organisations live in an increasingly aggressive and competitive environment.

- A very fast pace of change of technology is found at the productive level of society, faster than the pace of change found in management structures and regulatory rules.

- A high degree of integration and tight coupling of systems - one single decision can have dramatic effects that propagate rapidly and widely through the global society.

- An increasing scale of industrial installations with a corresponding potential for large-scale accidents. A very low probability of accidents has to be demonstrated to have operation accepted by society.

This situation has quite naturally led to an increased public concern about industrial safety and pressure groups have been very active, in some areas leading to a 'zero accident' concept and a call for effective, proactive risk management instead of reaction to past accidents.

During the recent decade this concern has also encompassed the medical field and less successful patient treatment has increasingly been attributed to 'human errors' on the part of people taking part in the dynamic flow of events, that is, doctors and nurses. Therefore, some observations on the conditions of risk management in the medical domain can be added to this list:

-   The medical work domain is considerably less structured than the industrial installations for which most human error studies so far have been made.

-   Likewise, the fuzzy concept of 'health' and of 'normal' patient conditions gives an unreliable reference for judgment of 'error'. After the fact, it may be easy to find an alternative, more 'correct' treatment, which could not have been foreseen. As was the case for the Zeebrügge accident, it is very difficult for a decision maker to see the whole picture in advance.

- The trend toward legal actions and huge financial compensation claims appears to increase the cost of treatment by generating high insurance premiums. The consequence appears to be extensive use of 'preventive medicine', that is, the use of more clinical tests than are objectively required and reluctance on the part of surgeons to take any chances in order to prevent subsequent blame for misconduct. Who are the losers? Patients close to the risky end of the spectrum and those on the waiting lists?

- Installations, e.g., in operating theatres, appear to evolve by a bottom-up aggregation of the latest equipment offered separately by the suppliers, not from a top-down work analysis of the activities. Equipment design appears to be competition-centred rather than use-centered and human factors research appears to be a response to problems from the past, not part of a design for the future. This probably reflects the different constraints of industrial development and academic research.

A basic consequence of the fast pace of change and the tight coupling systems is that development of new systems by incremental change based on past experience will be ineffective. Increasingly, design must be based on models of those mechanisms of work systems that will shape behaviour in the future.

Adaptive Behaviour in Cooperative Work

This situation raises the problem of modelling adaptive socio-technical systems (Rasmussen, 1997), a problem that points to several basic systems research and design issues.

Organisations and cooperating teams basically serve to control the operation of a loosely coupled work system. The division of work and adoption of roles depend on the control requirements of the work system such as its relational structure and degree of internal coupling, its topography, the work load involved, the accessibility of information, the information traffic necessary for coherent operation and so on.

In other words, the functional requirements of the work system shape cooperative structures bottom-up by posing constraints on the division of work among groups and individuals. Additional formal constraints on division of work originate from legal requirements, safety regulations, union agreements and organisational rules of conduct. However, within the constraints on division and coordination of work posed from such sources, there are many degrees of freedom within which to arrange the detailed division of work and to structure its coordination.

As with choosing between work strategies, the dynamic shifting of boundaries between roles assumed by individuals can be used to resolve resource-demand conflicts and to match performance to individual preferences. The subjective criteria active in this adaptation will be very situation dependent and directly related to the particular work process, such as perception of differences in work load among colleagues, the amount of communication necessary among agents for coordination and subjective preferences for certain activities, etc. In consequence, the actual work organisation is a very dynamic, relational framework which changes continuously with work conditions. As we saw in the Clapham Junction case, the adaptation of role allocation and work coordination in response to local cost-effectiveness pressure can lead to severe consequences.

Rochlin *et al.* (1987) have studied the normal work practice onboard an aircraft carrier to explain its high reliability that they attribute to an effective dynamic adaptation of cooperative patterns to situational characteristics. In spite of the formal military rank organisation, they found a shift to an effective informal 'high-tempo organisation' during aircraft take-down. One clear characteristic of the high tempo mode is a kind of operational redundancy, that is, an ability of the individual actor to move in and provide for the execution of a task if the primary units falter. They also emphasise the importance of fringe-consciousness and an updated, tacit context awareness for a high cooperative reliability and found the high reliability on the flight deck depended on a decision/management redundancy in terms of internal cross-checks on decisions even at the micro level:

"Almost everyone involved in bringing the aircraft on board is part of a constant loop of conversation and verification taking place over several different channels at once. At first, little of this chatter seems coherent, let alone substantive, to the outside observer. With experience, one discovers that seasoned personnel do not 'listen' so much as monitor for deviations, reacting almost instantaneously to anything that does not fit their expectations of the correct routine."

During our studies of work in hospitals, for example to investigate if computer based patient records should be introduced for operation theatre planning, we observed many situations when this kind of subtle, implicit communication and coordination took place which would be difficult to support by computer systems.

In a dynamic work situation, much information is communicated through body language and by other non-verbal means. In a shared, dynamic context, the need for explicit communication is decreased and short-hand comments are loaded with information. In this situation, it is clear that communication of intentions becomes very important for resolving ambiguities and correcting mistakes, not to mention trusting information and advice. When mutually familiar decision makers are communicating to solve a problem, subtle differences in the way a question is asked is of definite importance for the answer. An x-ray film analyst gave us the example that when faced with a particular film, he knows pretty well what question will be asked by the diagnostician. The important information for him is how the question is phrased. This kind of context dependent focus of a question is normally communicated by non-verbal means, but has a drastic effect on the reliability of communication.

In the hospital context, we have also observed some important implications of 'natural' decision making (Klein *et al.*, 1994) similar to the aircraft carrier case: operation theatre planning takes place during conferences or meetings including doctors and nurses. A typical feature of a hospital we studied appears to be a kind of collective memory. No one individual has available all the relevant information about the individual patients, rather a 'collective memory' has this information. When treatment of an individual patient is planned, the context from previous considerations defines an elaborate knowledge background. If, at a meeting, an action is proposed which is not supported by the knowledge possessed by another member of the group, this will be voiced properly. If the situation is ambiguous, one member will very likely offer comments up-dating the context. This goes on until the context is properly established and decision can be concluded by the surgeon in charge without alternatives being explicitly mentioned. In other words, decisions emerge when the landscape (the representation of work constraints) is well enough shaped so as to let the water (behaviour) flow in only one proper direction. One important aspect of this cooperative conditioning mode of decision making is the built-in redundancy similar to that described by Rochlin *et al.* Several persons with different perspectives on the patient's situation will accept the result of the negotiation. Another important aspect is that during evolutionary completion of the context that ultimately defines the conclusion, subtle observations may be offered for the resolution of ambiguities which could not be retrieved by an explicit question because a proper search question could not be phrased. Likewise, these important pieces of information would not be offered outside this face-to-face encounter (for example, entered into a database) because only the specific context makes it worth mentioning.

Thus field studies clearly show that safety on aircraft carriers as well as in healthcare depends on effective adaptation of the behaviour of individuals and their cooperative patterns to subtle situational features. Such clever recovery strategies of expert teams can only be understood from careful studies of their actual practice during normal work. Another lesson is the importance of a functional redundancy during critical periods. Unfortunately, the drive of modern business managers toward cost effectiveness will very likely remove the basis for this dynamic redundancy. To quote Rochlin *et al.*:

"In the classical organizational theory, redundancy is provided by some combination of duplication (two units performing the same function) and overlap (two functional units with functional areas in common). Its enemies are mechanistic management models that seek to eliminate these valuable modes in the name of efficiency."

A System Oriented Approach to Modelling Organisational Behaviour

To create a basis for design of reliable organisation, we need a model of the adaptive behaviour of individuals and organisations in response to environmental pressure. Injuries, contamination of environment and loss of investment all depend on loss of control of physical processes capable of injuring people or damaging property. Safety, then, depends on the control of work processes so as to avoid accidental, harmful side effects. It follows that risk management is a control problem and the examples mentioned above demonstrate that this control function involves several levels of decision makers, including government, authorities, management and operating staff and thus involves a complex socio-technical system. This system is normally decomposed according to organisational levels, and these levels are traditionally studied separately by different disciplines, see figure 2.2.

Furthermore, research within each discipline usually has a 'horizontal' orientation across the types of technological hazard sources and it is difficult, if not impossible, to create a model of the social control function that is active for a particular hazard by integration of models developed separately by academic research. These models do not 'connect': they are developed for teaching novices of the different professions, not for the design of systems that support professional experts. For instance, management theories and organisational models developed at business schools tend to be independent of the substance matter context of a particular productive system.

For design of effective safety control strategies we need careful studies of the 'vertical' interaction among the levels of socio-technical systems with reference to the nature of the hazard sources they are intended to control.

Most present research efforts reflect an academic research approach. Normally, a system is modelled by structural decomposition into parts and elements that are studied separately. In the same way, the continuous 'flowing' behaviour of a system (and those acting within it) is modelled by decomposition of this flow into discrete events. Such behavioural decomposition is the basis for identification of activity elements in terms of tasks, decisions, acts and errors.

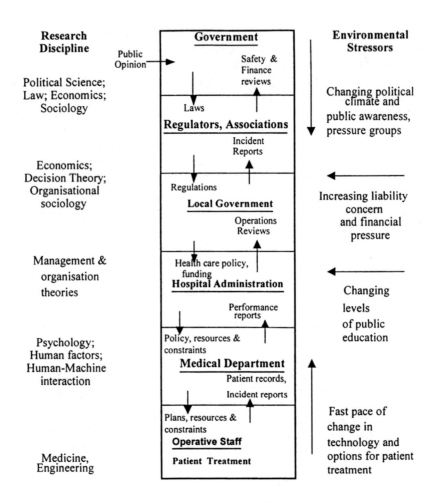

Figure 2.2. The socio-technical system involved in public healthcare. The upper levels control the policy, resources and constraints that constitute the pressure that may force the operative level toward the boundaries of safe operation. The various levels are normally studied separately by different research disciplines, having a *horizontal* orientation across hazard sources. The present paper argues for *vertically* oriented research considering the dynamic interaction among levels for particular types of hazards.

A fundamental problem with this approach is that all work situations leave many degrees of freedom of choice by the actors even when the objectives of work are fulfilled. To perform a task, these degrees of freedom will be resolved in the particular situation to find the 'path of least resistance', using subjective, situation dependent and often subconscious performance criteria, such as work load, time spent, or fear of failure. Consequently, for a dynamic and loosely structured work context such as healthcare, task performance changes significantly over time and a representation in terms of action sequences and errors is unreliable when studying actual performance during work. A representation in terms of task procedures is only relevant for highly constrained activities such as operation of technical equipment and even then many degrees of freedom are often left open. In general, therefore, no reference is found for judgment of errors in terms of a stable, correct practice.

MODELS OF ADAPTIVE SYSTEMS FOR DESIGN OF SAFER SYSTEMS

The conclusion of this discussion is that the design of a work support system in a modern, dynamic society cannot be based on 'task analysis' in terms of actions and errors.

Human behaviour in any work system is shaped by objectives and constraints which must be respected by the actors for work behaviour to be successful. Many degrees of freedom are, however, left open which will be closed by the individual actor in an adaptive search guided by local and subjective criteria such as work load, cost effectiveness, or risk of failure. Consequently, in a dynamic society, the design of work support systems based on models of work behaviour in terms of tasks, decisions, acts and errors is no longer a reliable approach.

We have to model work systems in terms of the mechanisms that generate behaviour in the actual, dynamic work context. That is, design must be based on an analysis of basic work requirements that define the functional structure of the work-space, the space of opportunities for action left to the actor's choice and the boundaries of safe operation. Furthermore, identification of the situational and subjective criteria serving the actual choice is important, together with an identification of the organisational and environmental pressures that will influence these criteria.

Therefore, one important research issue is to describe the interaction between the various levels of decision makers shown in figure 2.2 and to make explicit in the interfaces of their normal work support systems, the boundaries of safe operation and the impact of decisions on the constraints and decision criteria at the other levels. The trend toward use of integrated, computer based decision support systems makes such an approach possible, but we still need careful, vertically oriented studies within a particular work domain to define the information content of such a system.

At the lowest, operative level, some progress in this direction has been made by the design of 'ecological' interface displays that directly visualise the 'ecology of work', that is, the relational structure and the boundaries of safe operation. This approach has proven feasible for work systems that are reasonably well structured and can be explicitly described, such as process control and aviation (Rasmussen *et al.*, 1990; Vicente *et al.*, 1992; Rasmussen *et al.*, 1994, Flach *et al.*, 1995). Similar displays can probably also be developed for monitoring patients' circulatory systems. An example has been suggested to us in analogy to the displays developed for process control for monitoring the cardiac cycle. In this case, an integrated display based on the representation shown in figure 2.3 should replace presentation of several individual measurements and thus counteract the trade-off and the selection of under specifying cues, mentioned above.

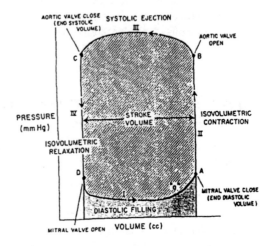

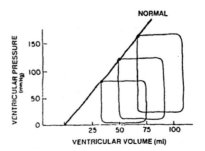

Figure 2.3. Monitoring the cardiac cycle by judging a set of measured variables during anesthesia is a complex task due to the complex relationship that defines normal circulation. However, this is directly visible from an integrated representation. The upper, left corner of the pressure-volume cycle should then follow a straight line, as shown.

At the higher levels of the socio-technical system we need the vertically oriented field studies to model the interaction in a way that will support design of improved visualisation for decision support systems. How do we assist the manager in visualising the impact of the resources available to, constraints upon and the decision criteria of actors at the operative level? How do we prompt his attention to decisions that will influence operational safety?

This approach points to a next phase of human factors based system design. Human factors and human computer-interaction research has recently focused on the *user-centered* approach, seeking to match the interface representation to the practice and mental models of experienced actors. However, evidence has since long shown that the mental models of users are unreliable outside the normal state of affairs (see, for example, Ackermann *et al.*, 1963). Therefore, the approach suggested here to cope with a dynamic environment is what John

Flach *et al.* (1992) has called a *use-centered* approach by which the interface is designed to represent the internal structure of the work environment and thus to create faithful mental models that support also response to a changing environment.

CONCLUSION

The conclusion of this discussion is that in order to increase safety and improve risk management in the medical field we have to leave the academic focus on task performance and errors observed in the past and turn to a study of the factors that create normal behaviour in the actual work system. This involves field studies in hospitals to create system based specification of equipment supporting Use-Centered design. It also involves studies of the constraints of the designers of equipment to improve communication with suppliers to influence their approach, which necessarily must be a Competition-Centred design. Academic critique of 'clumsy automation' on the part of 'stupid designers' misses the point. Only system-focused customer requirements can serve to merge the two approaches. Unless safety research can serve to shape the constraints of designers in a way leading to work systems that enforce safe behaviour, researchers are fighting windmills.

Unfortunately, research to create a basis for actual Use-Centered Design will be very cross-disciplinary, involving engineering, medical and cognitive psychology, an approach that poorly matches the constraints of a university environment. A solution to this problem has been suggested for public healthcare research by Kahn and Prager, 1994.

REFERENCES

Ackermann, W. and G. Barbichon (1963). Conduites intellectuelles et activite technique. *Bull. CERP* **12**, (1), 1-16.

Amendola, A. (1989). *Planning and Uncertainties*. Proceedings of the 2nd World Bank Workshop on Risk management and Safety Control. Rescue Services Board, Karlstad, Sweden.

Cook, R. I., D. D. Woods, and C. Miller (1998). A Tale of Two Stories: Contrasting Views of Patient Safety. National Patient Safety Foundation at the AMA.

Dominguez, C. (1998). Expertise in Laparascopic Surgery: Anticipation and Affordances. In: *Proceedings of Naturalistic Decision Making 4*. Warrenton VA.

Dominguez, C., J. Flach, D. McKellar and m. Dunn. (in press). The Conversion Decision in Laparascopic Surgery: Knowing Your Limits and Limiting your Risks. In: *Psychological Explorations of Competent Decision Making* (J. Shanteau, K. Smith and P. Johnson, eds.), Cambridge University Press.

Flach, J. M. and C. O. Dominguez (1995). Use-Centered Design: Integrating the User, Instrument, and Goal. *Ergonomics in Design*, July 1995, 19-24.

Hadamard, J. (1945). *The Psychology of Invention in the Mathematical Field*. Princeton University Press.

HMSO (1987). *M V Herald of Free Enterprise*. Her Majesty's Stationary Office, Report of Court, London

HMSO (1989). *Investigation into the Clapham Junction Railway Accident*. Her Majesty's Stationary Office, London.

Kahn, R. L. and D. J. Prager (1994). "Interdisciplinary Collaborations are a Scientific and Social Imperative." *The Scientist*, July 11, 12-13.

Klein, G., J. Orasanu, R Calderwood and C. E. Zsambok (eds.) (1994). *Decision Making in Action: Models and Methods*. Ablex, Norwood, NJ.

Mach, E. (1905). *Knowledge and Error*. English Edition: Reidel, 1976.

Paget, M. A. (1988). *The Unity of Mistakes. A Phenomenological Interpretation of Medical Work*. Temple University Press, Philadelphia.

Rasmussen, J. (1983). Skill, Rules and Knowledge; Signals, Signs, and Symbols, and other Distinctions in Human Performance Models. *IEEE Transactions on Systems, Man and Cybernetics*. Vol. SMC-13, No. 3, 1983.

Rasmussen, J. (1990a): Human Error and the Problem of Causality in Analysis of Accidents. *Phil. Trans. R. Soc. Lond.* B 327, 449-462.

Rasmussen, J. (1990b). Role of Error in Organizing Behavior. *Ergonomics*, **33**, nos 10/11, 1185-1190.

Rasmussen, J. (1993a). *Market Economy, Management Culture and Accident Causation: New Research Issues?* Invited lecture; Proceedings Second International Conference on Safety Science. Meeting Budapest Organizer Ltd, Budapest.

Rasmussen, J. (1993b). Diagnosis in Action. *IEEE Transactions on Systems, Man and Cybernetics,* **23** (4), 981-993

Rasmussen, J. (1994). Risk Management, Adaptation, and Design for Safety. Invited contribution to: *Future Risks and Risk management* (N. E. Sahlin and B. Brehmer, eds.). Kluwer Dordrecht.

Rasmussen, J. (1997a). Risk management in a Dynamic Society: A Modeling Problem. *Safety Science* 27/2-3, 183-213.

Rasmussen, J. and K. J. Vicente (1990). Ecological Interfaces: A Technological Imperative in High tech systems? *International Journal of Human Computer Interaction* 2(2) 93-111.

Rasmussen, J. and Pedersen, S. Andur (1991). *Causal and Diagnostic Reasoning in Medicine and Engineering*. Contribution to the CEC Basic Research Action project MOHAWC. Workshop May 1991, Stresa Italy

Rasmussen, J. and A. M. Pejtersen (1994). Virtual Ecology of Work. In: *Ecology of Man-Machine Systems: A Global Perspective* (J. Flach, P. Hancock, J. Caird and K. Vicente, eds.). Lawrence Erlbaum, Hillsdale, NJ.

Rasmussen, J., A. M. Pejtersen and L. P. Goodstein (1994). *Cognitive Systems Engineering*. Wiley, New York.

Rees S. and G. Rodley, (eds.) (1995). *The Human Costs of Managerialism: Advocating the Recovery of Humanity*. Pluto Press of Australia, Leichhardt NSW.

Rizzi, D. (1990). *Complications in Anesthesia: An Overview*. Risø National Laboratory. Internal Report, Roskilde.

Rochlin, G. I., T. R. La Porte and K. H. Roberts (1987). The Self-Designing High-Reliability Organization: Aircraft Carrier Flight Operations at Sea, *Naval War College Review*, Autom 1987.

Selz, O. (1922). *Zur Psychologie des Productiven Denkens und des Irrtums*. Friederich Cohen, Bonn.

Star, S. L. and E. M. Gerson.(1986). The Management and Dynamics of Anomalies in Scientific Work. *The Sociological Quarterly*, **28**(2), 147-169.

Vicente, K. J. and J. Rasmussen, (1992). Ecological Interface Design: Theoretical Foundations. *IEEE Transactions on Systems, Man and Cybernetics*, **22**(4), 589- 607, July/August 1992.

CHAPTER 3

ANALYSIS OF HUMAN ERRORS IN ANAESTHESIA OUR METHODOLOGICAL APPROACH: FROM GENERAL OBSERVATIONS TO TARGETED STUDIES IN SIMULATOR

Anne-Sophie Nyssen, Department of Work Psychology, University of Liège, Belgium

In anaesthesia literature, accident analyses often classify accidents into three exclusive categories: human error, equipment failure or complication. In general, 60 % to 87 % of anaesthetic mishaps are attributed to human error (Chopra *et al.*, 1992; Cooper *et al.*, 1978; Gaba 1989; Vourc'h, 1983). Human error is defined by the criterion of 'performance which deviates from the norm'. This definition implies a well-structured task sequence performed in stable and predictable work conditions (Rasmussen, 1993). This is not the case in anaesthesia. Although anaesthesia is usually referred to as a procedure for putting the patient into an unconscious state so that the surgery is possible, the action of the anaesthetist is highly contextual; it lies within an evolving situation marked by a transformation of the patient's state and by the surgeon's actions. Consequently, the activities involved include high level cognitive functions such as dynamic control of the physiological state of the patient and adaptive decision making to the context. There are, therefore, analogies with other complex domains already studied by Work Psychology.

In a previous article (De Keyser and Nyssen, 1993), we compared the anaesthesia situation to the nuclear power plant situation. Emphasis was placed on the proliferation of monitoring apparatus and the evolution of the anaesthetist's task towards 'supervisory control' as described by Sheridan (1987): in today's OR, the anaesthetist supervises, detects and regulates the case essentially from electronic screens. But, unlike industrial systems, patients are not designed or built by humans. Consequently, while the number of potential problem situations in an industrial environment is, in principle, limited, well-known and predictable, the anaesthetist must face a wide variety of problems for which no rote-learned procedure is available. Under such conditions, the usual convention to define human error in relation to the norm is difficult to apply. Moreover, the classification of anaesthetic mishaps into exclusive categories appears irrelevant in a world in which humans, technology and organisation are more and more connected. Even when human error is directly involved, it is always possible to point to problems in the design, manufacture, installation, maintenance, or organisation of some part of the system (Wagenaar *et al.*, 1990; Reason, 1997). Understanding how this complex system poses demands on the anaesthetist and how the anaesthetist meets those demands, seems more important for the prevention and management of errors than statistical and epidemiological data. This goal requires specific techniques to collect and analyse data but also raises different technical problems for collecting them, for instance problems relating to the confidentiality of the data.

In this chapter, we will summarise the methodological approach we used in a safety research programme that has been ongoing for the past six years in the Department of Anaesthesia and Intensive Care Medicine, University Hospital of Liege, Belgium. We will examine how we moved from general observations of the work to more targeted studies in a simulator in order to get an insight into human performance issues. Our methodology comprises the following steps:

- on-site observations of work and preliminary data collection by retrospective interviews,
- on-line questionnaires on problem situations and organisation of Quality Conferences,
- laboratory research in a full scale simulator using video recording and self confrontation.

Each step offers different potential to collect and analyse data on human performance and is subject to different kinds of biases. It is not our goal here to develop in detail the results of the research. However, the way in which each step improves our knowledge on performance problems is illustrated by means of the case study that is presented later in the paper.

ON-SITE OBSERVATIONS OF WORK AND PRELIMINARY DATA COLLECTION BY RETROSPECTIVE INTERVIEWS

On-site observations of work and preliminary data collection by interviews were performed in order to obtain information on central elements of the activity in the work context, of the type and use of technology and of the problem situations encountered. The main aim was to get familiar with the work situation and to identify those aspects of the work that required further investigation.

Naturalistic observations (more than 200 hours) were conducted in eight out of seventeen of the surgery ward's operating rooms, selected on the basis of differences in working conditions (type of operation - duration - monitors available - length of service of the anaesthetist). These observations led to a phenomenological account of anaesthesia task and a list of general patterns observed in behaviour (Nyssen, 1990; De Keyser and Nyssen, 1993). Results comprise: (1) a general description of the task environment, (2) an activity analysis in domain terms (description of a general procedure of an anaesthesia case, identification of sequence of actions and duration and (3) an analysis of practitioner cognitive activities.

The cognitive analysis of the task as developed by Rasmussen (1987), Woods and Roth (1988), and Patrick *et al.* (1986), is presented as a hierarchical break-down into objectives, means and constraints which allow for a response to the practitioner's 'why do', 'what to do' and 'how to do'. The criticisms of this were numerous: normativity, absence of real formalism and associated grammar (Grant and Mayes, 1991), absence of response to the 'when to do', etc. Nonetheless, its heuristic value in the determination of task difficulties cannot be denied.

Figure 3.1 presents some elements, albeit incomplete, of the cognitive analysis of the anaesthetist's task. The cognitive demands are described here at a very general level in order to contain not only the intrinsic goals derived from the task (e.g. need to provide unconsciousness, need to abolish sensation of pain, etc), but also the extrinsic demands derived from the environment (e.g. economic, institutional, organisational pressures, etc) that influence human decision making.

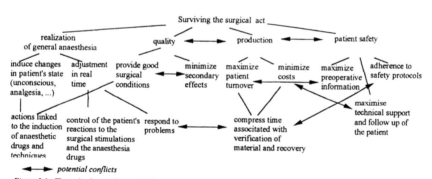

Figure 3.1 The task of general anaesthesia contains potential conflicting goals. For example, the production pressure may the anaesthetist to skip some steps in the procedure such as the verification of the material; some accute problem situations may require adoption of the protocol to the context; the goals of the surgeon and of the anaesthetist may differ in particvla situations and require negotiation.

Constructing this map cannot be done by reading textbooks of anaesthesiology or policy documents. It requires observation of what the practitioner actually does in his environment in order to construct a model of the contextual demands and understand the competing nature of some of them. With this model, the decisions and the actions of the anaesthetist take on new meaning: they often represent the optimum path to progress through the case, considering the local demands and the available means (De Keyser, 1989; Cook *et al.*, 1991).

After this first phase, a more systematic collection of data was installed: retrospective interviews were organised in order to collect a first sample of anaesthesia mishaps involving human error. One bias with retrospective interviews is posteriori justifications and rationalisations, especially in delayed interviews. The mode of questioning is crucial for collecting valuable data. We used the technique developed by Vermersch (1994), called the '*explicitation* interview', to avoid these bias. It is designed not to constrain the interviewer to one type of description during the interview and it gives cues to help him recall the global situation, avoiding rationalisations.

A first sample of 20 cases were collected from 12 expert anaesthetists using this technique. Diverse methodologies were applied to analyse the data. Among these, was the construction of a hypothetical causal structure for each case, conveyed graphically by a causal tree (Nyssen, 1990). This was to reconstitute the genesis of the incident and the conditions for production of human error.

The causal tree diagram was created in the 1970s by the Institut National Français de Recherche Scientifique (Krawsky *et al.*, 1981). It refers to the 'Failure Tree' method formalised by Bell Telephone and adopted by the aerospace industry. A number of researchers have used this technique in order to quantify human factors in reliability by calculating the probability of the occurrence of given events. One criticism often directed at this technique is that a causal tree based on a clinical method only provides a singular set of facts and circumstances. In spite of this limitation, a well-conducted clinical analysis remains a precious source of information.

A factorial analysis (Varimax rotation) carried out on this first sample allowed the identification of six factors associated with the 20 errors collected (Nyssen, 1997). These are:

- defaults in the management of information (mainly saturated by an absence of communication, difficult visibility and access to the patient, lack of adequate monitoring),
- inappropriate supervision (frame of mind of the novice with regard to the senior anaesthetist, late call for help, lack of experience, control of activity not continuous),
- productive pressure (saturated by organisational variables at the origin of rushing),
- multitasks in parallel (interruption and presence of a distracting element)
- cooperation problems (conflicts of authority, problems in interpersonal relationships between surgeon and anaesthetist in the face of an emergency or during the evolution of a case)
- constraints connected to the task (diversification of material, end of the week, fatigue).

These results agree rather well with those already found in the literature, notably by Gaba (1989). They bring out the importance of distractors which prevent the anaesthetist from realising that a change has come about in the patient's state and further, the quality of communication and coordination within the team. They also show that the temporal pressure tied to external synchronisers - for example, the hospital schedule - plays a role in the error while the temporal pressure ensuing from the seriousness of the patient's state does not have the same effect.

ON-LINE QUESTIONNAIRES ON PROBLEM SITUATIONS AND QUALITY CONFERENCES

The next stage of our methodological approach was to organise an on-line collection of problem situations in the work place in order to increase the study of concrete problem situations and to propose a framework for analysing them. Two tools were established: Quality Conferences and questionnaires.

Quality Conferences have been introduced as a regular teaching tool in the Department of Anaesthesia and Intensive Care Medicine. This practice has been in use for years in English speaking hospitals but is still uncommon in Belgium. The conference is based on voluntary reporting of critical events using a reporting form. Each volunteer is then invited to present the case to his peers within the month it occurred. These conferences played a crucial role in our methodology. They allowed us to appreciate the degree of adaptation of human performance to the context through the flow of communication between staff anaesthetists and residents.

The reporting form was formulated in order to gather individual information for each problem situation presented during these conferences. It was to be filled out as soon as possible after the incident by the anaesthetist involved.

Most accident reporting forms used by previous studies on risk in anaesthesia included: data of the patient with appreciation of the risk (ASA Physical Status), type of surgery, detailed anaesthesia procedure from premedication to recovery and even post-operatively, detailed report of the incident and appreciation of the associated factors. Although this information on what we term 'extrinsic' factors is the most objective way of collecting information about critical events, it may not be sufficient when proposing an accident reduction strategy considering the cognitive demands that the evolution of the anaesthetist's task place on human performance. For this reason, in our study, we complemented classical accident analyses based on the external factors with a cognitive analysis based on the decision functions involved in the event.

Labels for cognitive activities involved in the decision making process were created using the well-known Rasmussen's model of decision making (1986). This model subdivides the decision making sequence into at least four stages, (1) detection of the course of the event underway, (2) identification of the problem (hypothesis formulation), (3) evaluation of the priorities and (4) planning and execution of the intervention. Although this representation of decision making is still simplistic, its value for determinin of task difficulties cannot be denied. Many psychologists have used it to analyse human error in natural settings. We have used it to explore mental activities that could shape anaesthesia critical events in significant ways. Table 3.1 shows the proposed framework based on the Rasmussen's model of decision making being used in our reporting form. Three main phases of evaluation have been differentiated: preoperative anaesthetic risk evaluation, inadequate perioperative management and postoperative risk evaluation, the better to reflect the sequential structure of an anaesthesia case.

TABLE 3.1

Distribution of the critical decision functions to the situation, according to degree of training of the anaesthetist involved. For one problem situation, there can be several critical stages; thus the number of responses is not equal to the number of problem situations analysed.

	Anaesthetist Year of Training					
	N	2nd	3rd	4th	5th	Senior	Mixed
Failure to perceive information	13	3	4	3			3
Inappropriate pre. Evaluation	11	2	3	1	2	1	2
Failure to follow procedure	10	4	4	1	1		
Inadequate perioperative management	9	3	3	1			2
Difficult diagnosis process	8	2	4	1		1	
Inappropriate post. Risk evaluation	5		2	1	1		1

Although data collection is still going on, some preliminary analyses based on a sample of 30 cases reported during a period of 16 months are available (Nyssen et al., 1999). The distribution of the critical decision functions for the problem situation are listed in table 3.1. The results revealed that the critical phase in the decision making process is far from always the diagnosis. Most often cited was failure to perceive information during surgery. This concerned situations where either the anaesthetist did not detect some valuable information about the problem or detected it too late (for instance, bleeding, ischemia and airway obstruction). Analysis of our data also revealed different cognitive difficulties with different degrees of expertise. We observed that diagnostic difficulties were mainly experienced by anaesthetists in their 3rd year of training. This analytical perspective is interesting if we want to predict those cognitive failures connected with some particular work conditions (prototypical risk situations) and limit the risk through such means as training, or technical or organisational improvements.

LABORATORY RESEARCH ON A FULL SCALE SIMULATOR USING VIDEO RECORDING AND SELF CONFRONTATION

Field research is an important contributor to complex human performance studies. However, one limitation is that the researcher needs to have a profound knowledge of the domain to be able to examine the study critically. A typical failure is to get lost in the language of the domain. Another problem comes from the fact that experimental frameworks for testing specific hypotheses are difficult to organise in the field because of the variability and uncertainty of the work. Full scale simulators provide the possibility for this experimental setting. One advantage is that they allow prospective and repeated observations assisted by audio and video recording, but a limit is that the subject may be less implicated than in real work situations.

In our study, we used a full scale anaesthesia simulator to better understand the precise nature of anaesthetist decision making expertise. We compared and analysed the ways anaesthesia trainees, with varying degrees of experience, acted in 4 simulated problem scenarios: (1) heart rhythm troubles on the ECG, (2) myocardial ischemia[1], (3) anaphylactic shock[2], (4) malignant hyperthermia[3].

The simulator system used is part of the CASE Series: Comprehensive Anaesthesia Simulation Environment, built by CAE LINK Corporation (Binghamton, NY, USA), under a license with Stanford University. It has been used for the past three years by the Departments of Anaesthesia and Resuscitation of the University of Liège, the University of Louvain and the University of Brussels in the framework of a training program in crisis management (Gaba et al., 1994) with the collaboration of the Department of Work Psychology at the University of Liège.

It is presented in the form of a conventional operating room equipped with all the necessary equipment for an operation but where the patient has been replaced by a manikin best representing the clinical reality. Each simulation session is carried out in three phases : (1) a briefing during which information is given as to the outcome of the session and on the medical records of the patient (approximate duration 15 min.); (2) a simulation session of which the duration varies, according to the type of scenario, from 30 to 60 min. This session is recorded on video; (3) a debriefing during which the videotape is shown and the performance discussed (approximate duration 35 min.). We used MacShapa software (Interactive Software Environment for Protocol analysis, Sanderson 1993) to transcribe video data. It was designed to increase the interaction levels for visualising data, performing different types of analysis and developing an encoding language.

---

1. Changes of the ST segment of the ECG from the isoelectric level, leading to a ventricular fibrillation.
2. Immediate allergic reactions involving a generalized response to certain medications used by the anesthetist.
3. Lethal disorder of skeletal muscle metabolism triggered by volatile anesthetics or muscle relaxants.

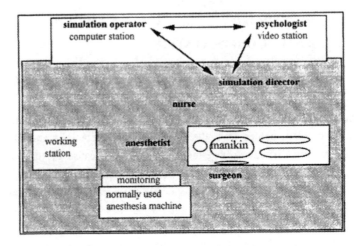

Figure 3.2 - Components of the full scale Anaesthesia Simulator (Belgium)

We used video recording of the performance to have access to the dynamics between the human performance and the problem context. Conducting such analysis in the real world is difficult because critical incidents are either uncommon or perceived as a unique occurrence. Video recording was also a very good medium for us to use in self-confrontation. With this support, subjects have much easier access to the thoughts they had during the simulation. The video supports not only the recall of the subject's decision making process, but also his or her understanding of the context in which it takes place.

During self-confrontation, we used an expert anaesthetist to provide evaluation of the quality of the trainee's performance and an expert psychologist to observe and code the trainee's behavioural responses. This interdisciplinary monitoring was crucial to understanding performance in a complex domain such as anaesthesia.

In order to characterise this performance, we used several performance indicators derived from our previous analysis of activity in the field study. These are: detection of relevant symptoms, hypothesis-driven searching and testing and specificity of the treatment undertaken.

We observed that the majority of the novices correctly diagnosed scenario 1 and scenario 2 but were unable to identify scenarios 3 and 4, while the more experienced anaesthetists handled this well. Data demonstrate that diagnosis times are shorter in the more experienced group.

The novice subjects stated more hypotheses than the more experienced subjects. The number of hypotheses does not only concern the ones verbalised by the subjects. Several studies have pointed out the difference in the verbalisations between experts and novices (Brinkman, 1990). The explanations given during the debriefings allowed us to infer, based on behavioural traces, the non-verbalised hypotheses underlying the actions of the more experienced anaesthetists. In scenarios 3 and 4, arriving at a correct diagnosis of the problem depends critically on the continued search for a solution following no improvement after initial corrective measures have been observed to have no effect. Novice trainees are able to evaluate the effect (or the non effect) of the treatment, as shown by comments, such as, "he is not responding to the perfusion", or "the situation is not improving", etc., but this evaluation of the situation does not seem to have the value of hypothesis testing.

These results shed light on the special abilities that experts possess that enable them to respond to problem situations, providing valuable information for a more realistic model of problem solving activities and consequently for developing criteria to assess whether proposed training programmes or technology developments will work sympthetically with the cognitive functions of the practitioner under a range of working conditions (Nyssen and De Keyser, 1998).

AN EXAMPLE OF OUR ANALYTICAL PROCESS

Let us present a case report to illustrate how different methods can improve our knowledge of performance problems.

> The anaesthetist on duty was scheduled to be on call that night. It was the beginning of the afternoon. The intervention was carried out on a two-year old child. The anaesthetic was administered without any problem and the surgical act finished. Hurried by the hospital planning, the anaesthetist extubed a bit too fast at the first signs of awakening (cough in the tube). The child went into a laryngeal spasm (the reflex closing of vocal chords causing a complete or partial glottal obstruction). The anaesthetist succeeded in quickly reintubing the patient and recovering the incident.

Because no harm actually came to the patient in this case, no trace of such a case would be found in most institutions, unless systematic collection (e.g. for Quality Conferences) was in effect. It seems (and seemed to peer experts who evaluated the incident in Quality Conferences) that the failure here consists of a poor evaluation of the patient's awakening state. It may seem simpler merely to attribute this case to human error and stop here. However, formulation of a causal tree reveals a more complicated story about human performance (Fig. 3.3). Moving back through the tree, it can be seen that there are more events linked to the organisation of work and fewer events linked to the anaesthetist's actions. Certain events constitute latent states present within the organisation before the incident, others are active errors. It is through their interaction that the problem situation arises.

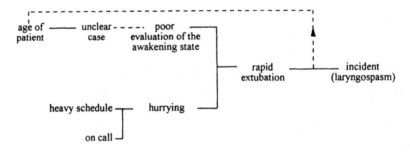

Figure 3.3 Hypothetical causal structure of incident

This incident also reveals the importance and the difficulty associated with the decision as to when to act. There are a number of events that must be synchronised when conducting an anaesthesia, notably because of the collective nature of the work. For instance, extubation must be carried out as soon as the surgical act is finished, when autonomous respiratory function is completely recovered, otherwise the risk of laryngospasm is increased.

Field observations are very important to gain access to the temporal structure of the task sketched in Figure 3.4 that constrains decision making. In this case, the misunderstanding of the patient's state was influenced by two factors:

i) the fact that the operation was on a child, a case in which observable parameters of the patient's respiratory function can lead to misinterpretations. Small children are known to fall back to sleep after the first signs of awakening; the anaesthetist must wait for this phase to pass before extubing the child.

ii) the competition between synchronisation constraints: the anaesthetist is simultaneously involved in several process of synchronisation. To a certain extent the hospital schedule inclines the anaesthetist to take risks: hence, the anaesthetist no longer waits until the end of the surgical act to decrease the drugs before extubing the patient, but anticipates it. With experience, he has learned to perceive the temporal relations of his work environment, to order events and to use them as 'Temporal Reference Systems' (TRS, Nyssen and Javaux, 1996) for an automatic and rapid mode of synchronisation. In this way, he reduces the awakening time and assures the synchronisation constraint linked to the hospital schedule. The success of the use of this synchronisation strategy depends on an invarient work situation; an unusual patient's condition can make this acquired strategy inappropriate and lie at the source of synchronisation failures.

Information support for the TRS used by the operators can be imagined as a means to help synchronisation activities. It is, however, absolutely necessary, to test the hypothesis of the TRS. Experiments on a simulator can be designed to lead to a thorough understanding of the synchronisation strategies and how to use this knowledge in operationally effective ways.

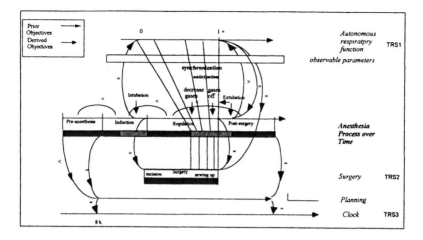

Figure 3.4 The experienced anaesthetist no longer waits until the end of the surgical act to decrease the drugs before extubing the patient, but anticipates it.

Conclusions

The driving idea beyond this chapter is that there is a need to use a wide set of research methods to get an insight into human performance in complex environments such as anaesthesia, where there are no operationalised expertise levels, no single correct answer to problems and where the observation and the measurement of real-world performance in a range of working conditions is difficult. The examination and re-interpretation of findings coming from various sources provide an insight. Each new finding provided by a specific method can point to different directions for improvement in safety (work practice improvement, training innovation, new technology development). These directions are not exclusive. Rather, they need to be coordinated in order to cover all the human performance issues relevant to safety in a large organisation.

1. The field observations reveal the complexity of the system in which practitioners work. They emphasise the system issues when studying human performance. The research results provide insight into how the system works, how the system (including regulatory, administrative and organisational factors) influences the decision of the practitioners and how it contributes to failure. In our experience, field studies are not only a method for gathering data on human performance in context but also a starting point for instituting a change in safety culture within the organisation. The presence of a researcher in the field provides a means to discuss safety and performance problems.

2. Generating systematic incident reporting and analysis is central to the continuing process of enhancing a change in safety culture. It requires a substantial effort from the practitioners, the teams, the department and the organisation. Many health care institutions have adopted the system of Quality Assurance Conferences based on voluntary reporting of

critical events. The success of this practice depends on how the analysis of the cases is conducted during the conferences in order to encourage people to voluntarily provide information. It is our belief that an inter-disciplinary collaboration between domain experts and psychologists is of value to guide the discussion in order to collect valuable information. In our study, we complemented classical accident analyses, based on the external contributory factors, with a cognitive analysis, based on the decision functions involved in the problem situation. The results of these analyses can be used to alert the department to the potential for some prototypical risk situations in order to reinforce the defensive filters to them.

3. Experimental studies shift attention away from the organisational context of the incidents and toward the human performance issues relevant to expertise. The goal of our study was to provide insight into the effectiveness of anaesthetist's education. First, we studied what makes problems more or less difficult for anaesthetists of different training levels by tracing the process of how they handle different problem situations in a full scale simulator. This helped us to identify the cognitive demands of problem solving, the strategies used and the critical information processing for the trainees (anticipation, task management, diagnosis testing). Finding results of this kind led us to reflect upon the means to enhance expertise, for example by the design of training objectives or by the development of decision aids that can effectively support practitioner cognition in the work situation.

The combination of methods described represents an active research process ranging from field situations to experimental situations. This movement promotes the enhancement of our knowledge on the role of human performance in complex dynamic situations. Only this knowledge will make it possible to go beyond the attribution of safety problems to the practitioners.

This research process is expensive to conduct and time-consuming for participants. It requires a long-term collaboration between the researchers and the practitioners. Ultimately, a scientific basis is created which can become the starting point for discussing and improving safety effectively in a given domain.

Figure 3.5 illustrates schematically the system model for safety we have formulated through this chapter. On the left of the model are the analysis perspectives of the work we combined. Each of the four levels can be provided by means of various methods. Examination and integration of the results provide information and knowledge on performance and expertise that can be used to select and design fine-tuning performance supports. Beside this level is the level of the integrated application of the solutions into the domain. Finally, on the right is the assessment of the effectiveness of the solutions. Because it offers an integrated mechanism for safety, we believe that this integrated model has a good potential for creating a 'positive safety culture' within an organisation which stimulates a variety of research methods and applications that actually improve safety.

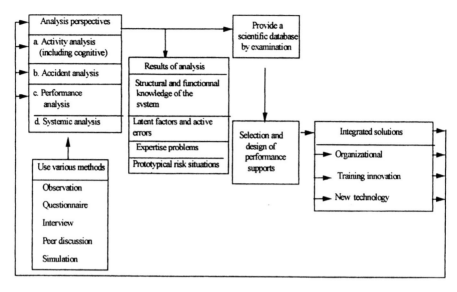

Figure 3.5 An integrated system model for performance and safety problems in complex environments.

REFERENCES

Brinkman, J. A. (1990). *The analysis of fault diagnosis task. Do verbal reports speak for themselves?* Unpublished doctoral dissertation, Technische Universiteit Eindhoven, Eindhoven.

Chopra, V., J. G. Bovill, J. Spierdiyk and F. Koorneef (1992). Reported significant observations during anaesthesia: a prospective analysis over an 18-month period. *British Journal of Anaesthesia*, **68**, 13-17.

Cook, R., D. Woods and J. McDonald (1991). *Human Performance in Anesthesia: A Corpus of Cases*. CSEL Report, Ohio State University, Columbus, USA.

Cooper, B., R. S. Newbower and C. D. Long (1978). Preventable anesthesia mishaps: a study of human factors. *Anesthesiology*, **49**, 399-406.

De Keyser, V. (1989). L'erreur humaine. *La recherche* . **216**: 144-1455.

De Keyser, V. and A.S. Nyssen (1993). Les erreurs humaines en anesthésie. *Le travail humain*, **56**, 233-241.

Gaba, D. (1989). *Causes of anesthetic mishaps: the problem of human error*. Rapport de recherche. Palo Alto.

Gaba, D., K. Fish and S. Horward (1994). *Crisis management in anesthesiology*. Churchill Livingstone, New York.

Grant, S. and T. Mayes. (1991). In: *Human Computer Interaction and Complex Systems* (G. Weir and J. Acty, eds.), Academics Press, Glasgow.

Krawsky, G., M. Monteau and J. Szekely (1981). La Méthode I.N.R.S. d'Analyse des Accidents, Outil de Gestion de la Sécurité. *Psychologie du travail*, **13**, 34-48.

Nyssen, A. S. (1990). *La fiabilité humaine en anesthésiologie. Recueil de cas - analyse approfondie - mesures de prévention*. Mémoire de fin d'études (unpublished), Université de Liège, Liège.

Nyssen, A. S. (1997). *Vers une nouvelle approche de l'erreur humaine dans les systèmes complexes : exploration des mécanismes de production de l'erreur en anesthésie*. Thèse de doctorat (unpublished), Université de Liège, Liège, Belgium.

Nyssen, A. S. and D. Javaux (1996). Analysis of synchronization constraints and associated errors in collective work environments. *Ergonomics*. **39**, 1249-1264.

Nyssen, A. S. and V. De Keyser (1998). Improving Training in Problem Solving Skills: Analysis of Anesthetist's Performance in Simulated Problem Situations. *Le travail humain* , **64**, 387-401.

Nyssen, A. S., E. Faymonville and M. Lamy (1999). Analysis of 23 critical events involving relatively healthy patients (submitted).

Patrick, J., P. Spurgeon and A. Shepherd (1986). *A Guide to Task Analysis: Applications of Hierarchical Methods*. An Occupational Service Publication, Birmingham.

Rasmussen, J. (1986). *Information processes and human-machine interaction: An approach to cognitive engineering*. North Holland, Amsterdam.

Rasmussen, J. (1987). *Modelling Action in Complex Environments*. Technical report Riso-M-2684, Riso National Laboratory, Roskilde, Denmark.

Rasmussen, J. (1993). Analysis of the tasks, activities and work in the field and in laboratories. *Le travail humain*, **56**, 133-147.

Reason, J. (1997). *Organizational Accidents: The management of Human and Organizational Factors in Hazardous Technologies*. Cambridge University Press, Cambridge, England.

Sanderson, P. (1993). *MacSHAPA* version 0.3 manual. Dept. of M & I.E.Urbana, IL.

Sheridan, T. B. (1987). In: *Handbook of Human Factors* (G. Slavendy, ed.), pp. 1243-1267. John Wiley & Sons, New-York.

Vermersch, P. (1994). *L'entretien d'explicitation*, ESF.

Vourc'h, G. (1983). Enquête épidémiologique sur les anesthésies. *Ann. Fr. Anesth. Réanim.*, **2**, 333-385.

Wagenaar, W., P. Hudson and J. Reason (1990). Cognitive Failures and Accidents. *Applied Cognitive Psychology* , **4**, 273-294.

Woods, D. and E.M. Roth (1988). Aiding Human Performance: II from Cognitive Analysis to Support Systems. *Le travail humain*, **51**, 139-171.

ACKNOWLEDGEMENTS

This work was supported by the Fond National Belge de la Recherche Scientifique and by the Politique Scientifique Belge (Programme de Santé du travailleur and PAI). We would especially like to thank Professor Lamy, M. L. Faymonville, M. Janssens and R. Larbuisson from the Department of Anaesthesia and Intensive Care of the University Hospital of Liege.

CHAPTER 4

CRITICAL INCIDENT REPORTING. APPROACHES IN ANAESTHESIOLOGY

Sven Staender, Department of Anaesthesia and Intensive Care, Kreisspital, Maennedorf, Switzerland

Mark Kaufmann, Daniel Scheidegger, Department of Anaesthesia, University of Basel, Basel, Switzerland

INTRODUCTION

Patient Safety in Anaesthesia: Medical Error in General

Clinicians working in modern anaesthesia departments perform a highly specialist task within a team. With the help of sophisticated equipment, surgery can now be performed on sicker patients than in the past. Surgery is often performed against a backdrop of stressful working conditions, for example high workload, intense time pressures, staff shortages and long working hours. Yet there is a requirement from surgeons, patients and society to achieve a high level of safety. Because anaesthesia practice is facilitative rather than therapeutic, there is very little tolerance for complications. Patients, relatives, surgeons and society expect that no patient should be harmed by anaesthesia care. This expectation has led to a steadily increasing awareness amongst anaesthetists of medicolegal and safety issues.

During the past four decades there has been a dramatic reduction in mortality caused by anaesthesia. Although there are few directly comparable studies, the trend is clear. The rate of death due to anaesthesia alone has been reduced from 1:1500 in studies covering the years 1957 - 1966 (Harrison, 1968) to about 1:150 000 in the late 1980s (Lunn and Devlin, 1987). Despite these encouraging developments, some issues merit close observation. We invest huge amounts of money on technical devices to increase safety, but on the other hand, there has been a tendency to neglect the important part played by human factors in error causation. This is a problem also seen in other high-risk working systems such as aviation.

This neglect is in strong contrast to the established finding that, in anaesthesiology, the leading cause of problems is human error. This was described as long as 20 years ago (Cooper *et al.*, 1978). Two important remarks are necessary at this point:

1. Despite the acknowledgement of the role of human error, specialists and society in general still do not yet accept error in the medical environment. Lucian Leape stated:

   "In everyday hospital practice, the message is clear: mistakes are unacceptable. Physicians are expected to function without error, an expectation that physicians translate into the need to be infallible. ... This kind of thinking lies behind a common reaction by physicians: How can there be an error without negligence?" (Leape, 1994).

   This approach forms the basis of professional education: the goal is error-free performance by medical professionals and we respond to failure by blaming individuals. This is not only highly unrealistic, it also prevents open discussion of errors in healthcare. Errors certainly occur and certainly will continue to occur, since human performance will always have its limitations.

2. Analysing errors (not only in healthcare) often leads to blaming individuals. But human factors specialists have discovered that many human errors have their roots in the system. Too often, analysing errors stops at the individual level, blaming the fallibility of the human being instead of looking for factors that might have impaired the performance level of this individual. Reason (1990) introduced the term of latent failures, describing circumstances in any system that sooner or later will lead to errors committed by the users of the system, namely the practitioners at the 'sharp end' working under these conditions, for example, doctors and nursing staff. These latent failures are often well beyond the control of individuals at the sharp end. In the medical domain these latent failures can be lack of standardisation, excessive reliance on memory, inadequate information available and poor working conditions. Any system that completely relies on human performance to function without error will fail, simply because humans are incapable of perfect performance.

Different Approaches to Evaluating System Safety

If we accept the fact that failures exist in everyday practice in hospitals we need to decide which method to choose to investigate these errors. Existing methods for error detection include: direct observation, chart reviews and/or computer screening, focus groups and incident reporting (Leape, 1997). All of them have advantages and disadvantages. In direct observational systems the main problem lies in the perception of those being investigated. Do practitioners accept a risk manager as a team member who helps them to increase their performance or is he perceived as a 'big-brother' figure watching over them?

Chart review and computer screening also rely on practitioners documenting correctly and not hiding potentially critical information that might endanger their career. Furthermore, charts have to be complete (much potentially dangerous practice may not be documented) and computer systems have to be implemented. Both chart review and computer screening furthermore require large-scale expenditure of both time and money.

Clinical focus groups can offer valuable information on risk in clinical practice. With a non-punitive approach and proper leadership, these meetings can facilitate discussions on safety limits, thus enlarging the safety margin of the operation under discussion. Voluntary reporting of critical events is another means to gain insight into dangerous situations. But incident reporting has its strengths and weaknesses. In the following we discuss these incident reporting systems further, with the help of two established systems, one in aviation and one in anaesthesia, before describing our own approach.

DEVELOPMENT OF THE CRITICAL INCIDENT TECHNIQUE

The technique of critical incident analysis was first introduced by Flanagan in 1954 (Flanagan, 1954). It was "an outgrowth of studies in the Aviational Psychology Program of the United States Army Air Forces in World War II", but has since been used in a variety of different ways. The aviation domain in particular has used this technique to overcome safety problems both in military and civil aviation. One result of these activities has been the implementation of a critical incident reporting system in the United States, the Aviational Safety Reporting System (ASRS). The system is operated by NASA and is largely funded by the US Federal Aviation Administration (FAA). The ASRS collects, analyses and responds to voluntarily submitted aviation safety incident reports in order to lessen the likelihood of aviation accidents. Pilots, air traffic controllers, flight attendants, mechanics, ground personnel and others involved in aviation operations submit reports to the ASRS when they are involved in, or observe, an incident or situation in which aviation safety was compromised. All submissions are voluntary and reports sent to the ASRS are held in strict confidence. ASRS's report intake was robust from the first days of the programme, averaging approximately 400 reports per month. More than 300,000 reports have been submitted to date and no reporter's identity has ever been disclosed by the ASRS. ASRS anonymises reports before entering them into the incident database. Each report received by the ASRS is read by a minimum of two analysts. Their first mission is to identify any aviation hazards and flag that information for immediate action. Analysts' second mission is to classify reports and diagnose the causes underlying each reported event. Their observations and the original anonymised report are then incorporated into the ASRS's database.

The ASRS acts on the information these reports contain. It identifies system deficiencies and issues alerting messages to those in a position to correct them. It educates through its newsletter CALLBACK, its journal ASRS Directline and through its research studies. Its database is a public repository which serves the FAA's and NASA's needs and those of other organisations world-wide which are engaged in research and the promotion of safe flight.

Beneath ASRS there are now a variety of other systems in place. Among them are:

- BASI, the Bureau of Air Safety Investigation in Australia,
- EUCARE, the European Confidential Aviation Safety Reporting Network
- Other systems, often run by the individual airlines, like Swissair, Air Canada, or American Airlines, to mention only a few.

In medicine, and especially in anaesthesia, such activities do not have a broad acceptance. The first application of the technique of incident reporting in anaesthesia was in the field of ergonomics of anaesthetic equipment (Blum, 1971). Cooper then adapted this technique to uncover patterns of frequently occurring incidents in an anaesthesia department (Cooper *et al.*, 1978). The Australians were the first to start using the critical incident technique in a national plan. The Australian Patient Safety Foundation, formed in 1987 set up and co-ordinated the Australian Incident Monitoring Study (AIMS) as a function of this Foundation (Webb *et al.*, 1993), with 90 hospitals and practices initially joined the study. Participating anaesthetist were invited to report, on an anonymous and voluntary basis, any unintended incident which reduced, or could have reduced, the safety margin for a patient. Any incident could be reported, not only those which were deemed 'preventable' or were thought to involve human error. After analysing 2000 critical incidents it was found that aspects of 'system failures' constitute the bulk of the contributing factors, even though human error can be detected in about 80% of the analysed cases (Runciman *et al.*, 1993).

Reporting to AIMS is principally done by completing paper forms and submitting them for analysis to the Australian Patient Safety Foundation. This results in much bureaucracy and delays in the dissemination of the information on critical events among anaesthetists. At the Department of Anaesthesia at the University of Basel, Switzerland we have therefore set up an anonymous critical incident reporting system (CIRS©) for anaesthetists in 1996 based on standard Internet technology (Staender *et al.*, 1997). This system runs on the Internet, on our local net at the University of Basel and as a national incident registry again using the Internet but protected against undesired visitors by a firewall. Before we go into the details of CIRS, some general remarks on the technique of incident reporting, its requirements, strengths, and weaknesses follow.

UNDERSTANDING CRITICAL INCIDENTS

Definition of a Critical Incident

The question of how to define critical events in anaesthesiology and how to distinguish them from accidents is a continuing debate. In aviation, incidents are distinguished from accidents simply on the basis of not doing any harm to personnel (passengers and staff) and only minor damage to the equipment. The problem in the medical field lies in the very variable outcome of incidents. Many scenarios have a potential for a very serious outcome, but many ultimately only result in patient dissatisfaction, unplanned ICU admittance or some minor and temporary morbidity. One example is asystole following spinal anaesthesia where cardio-pulmonary resuscitation restores normal sinus-rhythm but results in a fractured rib. There was no other definite outcome apart from the fractured rib, but the potential outcome could easily have been death. Was the event an *accident* (the fractured rib) or *incident* (potentially life-threatening situation)?

In CIRS, we therefore decided to ask practitioners to report on events under anaesthetic care that have the potential to lead to an undesirable outcome if left to progress. We then individually decide during case analysis whether each individual report constitutes an incident or in fact would better be regarded as an accident. As in AIMS, it was decided to include all incidents, not only those which were deemed 'preventable' or were thought to involve human error. Furthermore, practitioners were ask to report every incident fulfilling this definition regardless how trivial they seemed.

Another difficulty in the evaluation of hazardous situations lies in the problem of having no real 'golden rules of practice' in anaesthesia or in medicine generally. In medicine, many different ways to practice and manage certain situations are feasible and appropriate. This creates further uncertainty on the question of what constitutes a critical event.

SYSTEMS REQUIREMENTS FOR SUCCESSFUL INCIDENT REPORTING

Confidentiality and Attitudes to Error

First of all, such incident reporting systems have to be confidential, in the sense that reporters must know that the submitted information will not be used against them. In a recent editorial, Cooper stated: "why should we expect clinicians to report their own adverse outcomes if reporting might jeopardise their career?" (Cooper, 1996). The presence of an independent organisation is also crucial: "The second requirement is for a respected body, one independent of the influences of other stakeholders, to conduct the collection and analysis of data." (Billings, 1998)

Once confidentiality is assured, cultural change is also necessary. This change must take place on two levels. The first is at the level of the professional culture, since doctors have highly unrealistic attitudes about their vulnerability to error. The second change must be effected at the level of the organisational culture and of the society. Organisations must recognise and publicly acknowledge the inevitability of human error and adopt a non-punitive stance toward error - not only at the individual's level but also at the system's level. The saying, "We must learn from our mistakes or be doomed to repeat them", captures the essence of error management in a blame-free organisation. Furthermore, this open-minded acknowledgement implies a strong potential for learning. "Human learning takes place through action. Trial-and-error defines limits, but its complement, trial and success, is what builds judgement and confidence. To not be allowed to err is not to be allowed to learn." (Rochlin, 1997).

Anonymity

Close to the condition of confidentiality lies the condition of anonymity. Although anaesthetists are extremely safety conscious, they fear legal punishment. Their anxieties must be kept in mind and taken seriously. Incident reporting systems should certainly not conceal unsafe acts that obviously should have legal implications, but incident reporting systems should enable anaesthetists to exchange their experience on potentially dangerous situations. Obviously, it would be very convenient to have the possibility to ask a reporter for further details of a certain incident. But, presently, the error-culture in medicine does not seem to be developed enough to allow discontinuation of the anonymous approach of such incident reporting systems.

Information Feedback

A much more friendly requirement of such incident reporting systems is the need to spread the received information on critical events. Users of such systems should not only be asked to submit their experience, but should also have an immediate benefit from participating. This is absolutely crucial if these systems (as we would very much suggest) are kept voluntary.

In CIRS© we give all the relevant information back to each user of the system. From this we hope to motivate people and show them what kind of cases are of interest for us. Information feedback therefore serves as a tool for continuous education, which facilitates discussion of these events and motivates users to also submit their personal experience. Methods for enhancing the use of voluntary reporting systems could therefore be:

- presentation of the clinical information of each case
- discussion of individual cases
- giving users the possibility of an expert-opinion on their own case
- having the potential to search for certain topics in the whole set of already reported events
- publishing trends and findings of extraordinary cases

This concept of information feedback probably is very important for motivation of the people at the sharp end to share their experience. In ASRS highly professional staff screen, analyse and publish the cases on a regular basis. Success certainly lies in the highly professional status of the analysts. A system administrated by clerks with no detailed knowledge of the involved profession would not be viable. But with this need for a 'first-class' feedback, high professional expertise has its price. In ASRS for example, the overwhelming number of some 35,000 to 40,000 reports a year enter the system. The costs needed to cope with this workload on a highly professional standard is about two million dollars per year (Billings, 1998).

Analytical Framework

After considering the implementation of such systems, the question of how to analyse such cases arises. Once we have agreed that the majority of error can be reduced to system failure, the appropriate question is: which kind of system failures exist? The common categories include failures of design (process design, task design and equipment design) and failures of organisation and environment (presence of psychological precursors such as conditions of the workplace, schedules etc., inadequate team building and training failures). Such a framework can help categorising and analysing critical events and errors significantly. Van der Schaaf established a model in the chemical process industry and extended this model to the medical domain (van der Schaaf and Shea, 1996b; van der Schaaf, 1996a). In confidential interviews he groups the causes of error of the reported cases into the following categories: technical, organisational, human and patient related. We believe, that the category of 'team' must be added to this system, especially in anaesthesia, where we very often work in teams and also sometimes fail in teams.

Categorisation and analysis are very important because failure is often seen as a unique event. Often individual cases are considered as an anomaly without a wider meaning for the domain in question. Especially in accidents, commentary typically emphasises how the circumstances of the accident were unusual and did not have parallels for other people, other groups, other organisations or technological systems. This sometimes results in the statement: we are more careful, we are more conscientious (Cook *et al.*, 1998).

GOALS OF INCIDENT REPORTING SYSTEMS

Contributing Factors and Recoveries (*root factor detection*)

By establishing systems to report on critical events in anaesthesiology we hope to gain insight into questions regarding contributing factors to unsafe conditions, causes of error, knowledge about rare but potentially dangerous situations and methods of recovery from incidents. The recovery aspect of incident analysis is particularly promising in our eyes since incidents in contrast to accidents allow the review of conditions that prevented the event becoming a catastrophe. "What saved the day?" is the appropriate question to ask when we want to learn what each individual or technique contributed to preventing a potentially dangerous situation progressing to a bad outcome. In accidents, this question can no longer be raised, since the worst outcome of this special event has already happened. However, we do not discount the analysis of deaths and non lethal complications, which continues to contribute to improvements in anaesthetic safety. But incident analysis has a great potential for gaining knowledge of positive safety contributions (and not only on failures) that is too often forgotten.

Contributing factors to critical incidents in anaesthesiology have already been studied in detail and human factors have been identified in about 80% of the cases (Cooper *et al.*, 1978). Further in-depth analysis or even root-cause detection using an anonymous reporting system requires an extensive questionnaire to ask for all the details that are necessary to perform this analysis. A proper root-cause analysis can probably only be done using the technique of detailed and structured interviews with the reporter of critical events, thus violating the concept of anonymity. It is probably not possible to identify all latent failures using an anonymous approach to reporting.

Exchange of Information on Rare Cases

Knowledge about rare but potentially dangerous situations is very easily spread using electronic media. In CIRS© for example the description, as well as information on the management and outcome of each reported incident, is provided to every user of the system. This forms a collection of cases that may be rare but nevertheless provides lessons even for experienced practitioners. Such information may also provide early warning of potential hazards of a new technology. One strong report of a critical incident may be needed to warrant action.

Extent of the Problem (estimation of baseline)

In well functioning systems, a long observational period as well as a series of cases could provide a baseline of a problem's frequency that could be observed over time (as a kind of trend monitor). Furthermore, changes in practice or policy could then be assessed for any influence on the margin of safety. But for these two goals of reporting, both a huge database and a high level of compliance are necessary. Monitoring of critical incidents can give these large numbers much earlier than looking for accidents, since reporting of incidents yields a much larger database compared to accident-reporting in a given amount of time.

Goals of Reporting in Local Systems Versus on a National Basis

In principle, all of the above stated general goals are achievable when such systems are run locally. Furthermore, knowledge of the local system, its policies and procedures helps in analysing the incidents. Running the same system on a national basis means asking for far more detail to accomplish the same goals, simply because the analyst does not know anything of the individual conditions. For a national system therefore it might be reasonable initially to have reports with an identified reporter in order to allow the administrator of the incident system to contact the incident-reporter. If necessary, the reporter can be asked for further details of the case, for certain contributing factors or even latent failures. But these systems must maintain complete confidentiality, otherwise we doubt that there will be much contribution on a national level. Being an independent organisation is probably one of the most important success factors for the aviation reporting system ASRS, especially since ASRS is operating with this principally non-anonymous, confidential approach.

STRENGTHS OF INCIDENT REPORTING

To summarise, the advantages of incident reporting, both local and national, are:
- Incidents happen far more often than severe accidents. Therefore, analysing incidents provides a far broader database in a given amount of time. "The objective of initial data collection is to obtain a stable and reproducible measure of the

problem in order to be able to determine the effect of an intervention." (Leape, 1997)

- The analysis of incidents gives the opportunity to look for recoveries out of dangerous situations. Such analyses cannot be carried out with accidents, simply because there is no recovery.

- Incident analysis can (under certain conditions) lead to the root-causes of errors. These detected root-causes can then form the basis of very effective quality-improvement actions.

- Tracking incidents allows a monitoring of the quality of the structure and process of certain endeavours over time and over change in policies, if compliance is high.

- Exchanging experiences on critical events has a significant teaching potential even for old professionals, thus empowering people and teams.

- Costs are low compared to other methods, provided the system is not implemented by a large, national organisation, such as the ASRS with a yearly budget of two million dollars (Billings, 1998). On a local level, incident reporting probably is good value for money, when you keep in mind that the patient care costs of a preventable adverse drug event were calculated at more than 4000 dollars (Bates *et al.*, 1995).

WEAKNESSES AND LIMITATIONS OF INCIDENT REPORTING

Underreporting

Underreporting and the lack of an appropriate denominator[1] is certainly a major handicap of voluntary reporting systems. There is evidence that we still face a huge underreporting of critical incidents. In a study of predefined critical incidents that were automatically detectable (blood-pressure drop or desaturations during anaesthesia), it was found that only 4% of the automatically detected events were voluntarily reported (Sanborn *et al.*, 1996). The same was true in a simulator environment where participants were exposed to critical events and encouraged to report their experience later in an incident reporting system. Even under these conditions an inaccurate reporting of critical events was found (Byrne and Jones, 1997).

---

[1] Denominator – the absolute number of times an event occurs.

Reasons For Not Reporting

A recent study by Vincent *et al.* looked for reasons of not reporting adverse incidents in two obstetrical units (Vincent *et al.*, 1999). The main reasons were fears that junior staff would be blamed, high workload and the belief that the circumstances or outcome of a particular case did not warrant a report.

Participants of this study recommended that for a successful reporting there should be:

- induction training for all clinical and nursing staff (permanent, locum and agency) on risk management and incident reporting
- continuing education on the aims and importance of risk management and incident reporting
- a clear statement that *all* members of staff, regardless of profession and grade, are responsible for reporting
- a clearly defined list of reportable incidents/indicators drawn up in consultation with medical and nursing staff and a clear definition of incidents and drug errors to be reported
- 'user-friendly' incident reporting forms
- clarity on how to report, whether in writing, by telephone, or in person to the risk manager
- encouragement for staff to report an incident even if they are unsure whether it is necessary to do so
- a designated person on each shift who is responsible for checking that any incident occurring during that shift is reported
- a Trust/Hospital policy of 'no blame' and no disciplinary action except in cases of gross misconduct, repeated errors despite retraining, or criminal negligence
- regular feedback to staff regarding the action taken as a result of their reports

Bias

Another problem with the anonymous character of such incident reporting systems lies in the inability to validate the submitted information and the possible bias of reporters using such systems. First, there can be some uncertainty about *who* is reporting and *what* gets reported (Stanhope *et al.*, 1999). Knowing the outcome of a certain case can also influence both the reporter and the analyst. Jayasuriya found that compliance with reporting was high with more serious events and poor in the case of common events, or when successful recovery had occurred (Jayasuriya and Anandaciva, 1995). When it comes to analysis, grading and evaluation of reported events, knowing the outcome also influences judgement. Caplan *et al.*

(1991) asked anaesthesiologists to judge appropriateness of care in 21 cases involving adverse anaesthetic outcome. The original outcome in each case was classified as either temporary or permanent. The authors then generated a matching alternative case identical to the original in every respect except that a plausible outcome of opposite severity was substituted. They demonstrated that knowledge of the severity of outcome influenced a reviewer's judgement of the appropriateness of care, in that quality of care was more harshly judged in cases with poor outcome.

This outcome bias is minimised in analyses of incidents as compared to accident evaluations, simply because there is no adverse outcome in the majority of incidents. This is another advantage of dealing with incidents instead of accidents. Keeping these limitations in mind, we nevertheless believe that certain trends can be detected from voluntary and anonymously reported critical incidents which can be used as the basis for action to improve safety.

The following table summarises the different approaches to incident reporting that exist.

TABLE 4.1

Overview of Different Systems for Incident Reporting

System characteristics	Strengths	Weaknesses
Anonymous, Voluntary, Confidential	• broad basis for acceptance even in systems with poor safety culture • baseline and trend observation • detection of safety hazards • easy to implement • low cost	• no root cause analysis possible • no denominator[1] available • reporting bias
Voluntary, Confidential	• root cause analysis • baseline and trend observation • detection of safety hazards	• dependent on error-culture for sufficient reporting • no denominator available • reporting bias
Mandatory, Confidential	• same as voluntary, confidential • approximation of denominator[1]	• risk of 'big-brother' approach

[1] *Denominator means the absolute number of events to which one can compare the observed numbers.*

IMPLEMENTATION

CIRS©, the Approach to Incident Reporting in Switzerland

The Department of Anaesthesia at the University of Basel serves as a unit in a teaching hospital. A staff of 24 fully trained and licensed anaesthesiologists, 40 residents and 40 nurse anaesthetists, covers some 17,000 anaesthetic cases per year. Due to the teaching requirements the spectrum of experience of the residents ranges from one year after medical school to fully trained anaesthesiologists. Every sub-speciality including anaesthesia for cardiac surgery and neurosurgery is represented. The safety standards of our department requires a team of two experienced practitioners to be at the patient site during critical phases of the procedure such as induction or emergence from anaesthesia 24 hours a day and 365 days a year.

CIRS© is implemented on the local network using Internet technology. It is protected with a strong firewall that satisfies the stringent legal requirements of the national data-security act. CIRS© can be reached from every networked computer in the hospital. Computers are located in the offices, the theatre, the recovery room and the intensive care unit. Therefore, participating in CIRS© is possible from very different locations within the hospital.

CIRS© is completely electronic. From a typical Internet page, several local links are possible: links to background information about the project, links to the questionnaire, links to previously reported cases and links to extraordinary cases with a great teaching potential. The content of the detailed questionnaire (HTML-form) is automatically inserted into a central database. This database provides the users with the above mentioned details of every case and allows an easy compilation of the data. Furthermore, with the help of a kind of dynamic, database driven bulletin-board, an anonymous discussion of each case is possible. CIRS© is now in its third year and we have already received some 200 cases.

Analysing 132 critical incidents showed that in 64% of the cases, human factors such as tiredness, haste, wrong decision making and reduced situational awareness contributed to the incident. Adding the factor of problems in team performance, namely insufficient communication, increased the rate to 83%.

On the other hand, in these 132 critical incidents, 167 recoveries were cited (more than one recovery per incident was possible). The principal types were:

- following rules and algorithms   7%
- good communication/team performance   31%
- human recovery (vigilance, experience) 46%
- technical aspects   16%

Adding team-performance aspects to all the other human recoveries shows that human safety contributed in 77% of the cases to a harmless outcome from an initially critical incident (in 90% of the cases the outcome was not affected by the event or lead 'only' to patient dissatisfaction or prolongation of hospitalisation).

Already some safety weaknesses have been detected and acted on. For example:

1. The local pharmacy provides us with locally produced drugs like Lidocaine, Mepivacaine and Calcium chloride. Unfortunately, the labelling of the ampoules of all three drugs was such that they could very easily be confused. After detecting this safety hazard in one incident report, the local pharmacy has established a colour-coding system, that should allow easier identification of each drug.

2. For many years the muscle relaxant drug Succinylcholine has been routinely prepared in the obstetric unit even for minor procedures in order to rapidly induce and intubate a patient if necessary. Having the drug already drawn up in a syringe led to its inadvertent use in a patient under local anaesthesia. A heavy workload and a dense scheduling of patients on that particular day contributed to the incident. Being muscle-paralysed and conscious is one of the worst scenarios in anaesthesia. In this case, the team reacted immediately and induced general anaesthesia. Therefore, the patient did not have to suffer for more than a few seconds. Nevertheless, this caused us to change our practice. From now on, Succinylcholine is still available nearby, but no longer already drawn up in a syringe.

In the second example, the primary cause of the incident was apparently human error. The practitioner chose the wrong drug. A closer look at this event demonstrates that the procedure (drawing up a potentially life-saving but also dangerous drug) has its pitfalls and that time-pressure and haste contributed to the evolution of this event. Therefore, two latent failures (dangerous protocols and the lack of staffing) caused this problem. A cursory analysis would grade this incident as human error related, whereas it is probably better regarded as a systems failure.

Since the end of 1998 we have also used this system as a tool for a national incident survey in anaesthesiology in Switzerland (CIRS©-CH). This national system operates under the auspices of the National Society of Anaesthesiology (SGAR) in order to facilitate reporting. Again, this system, also running on the Internet, is protected, accessible only after an individual login procedure. Therefore it cannot be visited from outside. A national board of experts from different regions of Switzerland and different classes of hospitals maintains this system, publishes the national results and acts as a facilitator for expert-opinion on selected cases. This feedback on individual cases was regarded as most important for national success. It is worth noting that the analysis and comments on the events require at least as much expertise as is involved in their generation. Furthermore, an international version of CIRS© now exists that is very similar to the local and national system. The unprotected international version of CIRS© is freely available on the Internet at: http://www.medana.unibas.ch/cirs/. This Internet-site offers insights into this system.

CIRS© is regularly scanned for certain extremely important cases that would require immediate action. Then, from time to time, summary statistics are performed and the findings published. An analysis of underlying causes of error can be done on the local level, where sufficient information about the system is available. On the national level, this root-cause analysis is not possible, simply because of the anonymity of the system and the limited amount of details in the questionnaire about the unit and environment the reporter works in. Nevertheless, we believe that the national exchange of information on critical events enhances patient safety in Switzerland.

SUMMARY AND POSSIBLE FUTURE DIRECTIONS

Incident reporting as a means of detecting safety deficits has strengths and limitations. Most incident reporting discussions revolve around how to achieve greater compliance with reporting requirements in order to gain more reports. We must perhaps accept the fact, that in voluntary systems (which we strongly recommend) there is huge under-reporting. Rather than discuss how to increase reporting, we should consider what kind of information can be derived from existing incident reporting systems such as AIMS, CIRS© or ASRS. What should we ask and how can we deal with the data reported.

"A central question facing us is not really how many there are, but how many is enough. That is to say, there are already many signals that point to a variety of failures. Part of the consensus that needs to be formed for successful incident reporting is consensus about what is a sufficiently strong signal to warrant action." (Billings, 1998).

We believe, that under certain circumstances and with all the limitations kept in mind, the voluntary and anonymous reporting of critical incidents in anaesthesiology can help to enhance safety in this speciality. Furthermore, if we detect certain recurring situations out of the reported cases, it definitely would be possible to feed these scenarios into anaesthesia simulators. Again, such training on rare events could be an important contribution to training and safety in anaesthesiology.

In future we want to expand our study of recoveries and successful management of critical situations. We should not only look for the weak aspects of systems but also for innovative activities that help practitioners to cope with the pitfalls of their daily work. In particular, we want to look for successful recovery-strategies instead of 'only' looking at the weak parts. We no longer want to blame the individuals, or certain systems, but instead look at strategies that empower humans at the sharp end to perform effectively in their systems.

REFERENCES

Bates, D. W., D. J. Cullen, N. Laird, L. A Petersen, S. D. Small, D. Servi, G. Laffel, B. J. Sweitzer, B. F. Shea, R. Hallisey and et al (1995). Incidence of adverse drug events and potential adverse drug events. Implications for prevention. ADE prevention study group. *JAMA* **274**, 29-34.

Billings, C., R. I. Cook, D. D. Woods and C. Miller (eds.) (1998). *Incident Reporting Systems in Medicine and Experience with the Aviation Safety Reporting System.* pp.52-61. Chicago, Il, USA: National Patient Safety Foundation at the AMA.

Blum, L. L. (1971). Equipment design and 'human' limitations. *Anesthesiology* **35**, 101-102.

Byrne, A. J. and J. G. Jones (1997). Inaccurate reporting of simulated critical anaesthetic incidents. *Br.J.Anaesth.* **78**, 637-641.

Caplan, R. A., K. L. Posner and F. W. Cheney (1991). Effect of outcome on physician judgments of appropriateness of care. *JAMA* **265**, 1957-1960.

Cook, R. I., D. D. Woods and C. Miller (1998). *A Tale of Two Stories: Contrasting Views of Patient Safety.* Chicago, Il, USA: National Patient Safety Foundation at the AMA.

Cooper, J. B. (1996). Is voluntary reporting of critical events effective for quality assurance? [editorial]. *Anesthesiology* **85**, 961-964.

Cooper, J. B., R. S. Newbower, C. D. Long and B. McPeek (1978). Preventable Anesthesia Mishaps: A Study of Human Factors. *Anesthesiology* **49**, 399-406.

Flanagan, J. C. (1954). The critical incident technique. *Psychol Bull* **51**, 327-358.

Harrison, G. G. (1968). Anaesthetic contributory death - its incidence and causes. Part 1. Incidence. *S.Afr.Med.J.* **42**, 514-518.

Jayasuriya, J. P. and S. Anandaciva (1995). Compliance with an incident report scheme in anaesthesia. *Anaesthesia* **50**, 846-849.

Leape, L. L. (1994). Error in medicine. *JAMA* **272**, 1851-1857.

Leape, L. L. (1997). A systems analysis approach to medical error. *J Eval.Clin.Pract.* **3**, 213-222.

Lunn, J. N. and H. B. Devlin, (1987). Lessons from the confidential enquiry into perioperative deaths in three NHS regions. *Lancet* **2**, 1384-1386.

Reason, J. (1990). *Human Error.* Cambridge University Press, Cambridge.

Rochlin, G. I. (1997). *Trapped in the Net: The unintended consequences of computerization.* Princeton University Press, Princeton, NJ.

Runciman, W. B., A. Sellen, R. K. Webb, J. A. Williamson, M. Currie, C. Morgan and W. J. Russell (1993). The Australian incident monitoring study. Errors, incidents and accidents in anaesthetic practice. *Anaesth.Intensive.Care* **21**, 506-519.

Sanborn, K. V., J. Castro, M. Kuroda and D. M. Thys (1996). Detection of intraoperative incidents by electronic scanning of computerized anesthesia records. Comparison with voluntary reporting. *Anesthesiology* **85**, 977-987.

Staender, S., J. Davies, B. Helmreich, B. Sexton and M. Kaufmann (1997). The anaesthesia critical incident reporting system: an experience based database. *Int.J Med Inf.* **47**, 87-90.

Stanhope, N., M. Crowley-Murphy, C. Vincent, A. O'Conner, and S. E. Taylor-Adams (1999). An Evaluation of Adverse Incident Reporting. *J Eval.Clin.Pract.*

van der Schaaf, T. W. (1996a). PRISMA: A Risk Management Tool Based on Incident Analysis. pp.242-251.

van der Schaaf, T. W. and C. E. Shea (1996b). MECCA: Incident Reporting Lessons from Industry applied to the Medical Domain.

Vincent, C., N. Stanhope and M. Crowley-Murphy (1999). Reasons for not Reporting Adverse Incidents: an Empirical Study. *J Eval.Clin.Pract.*

Webb, R. K., M. Currie, C. A. Morgan, J. A. Williamson, P. Mackay, W.J. Russell and W. B. Runciman (1993). The Australian incident monitoring study: an analysis of 2000 incident reports. *Anaesth.Intensive.Care* **21**, 520-528.

CHAPTER 5

A SYSTEMS APPROACH TO MEDICAL ERROR

Marilyn Sue Bogner, Institute for the Study of Medical Error, Bethesda, MD, USA

Risk and safety issues in medicine typically focus on serious adverse outcomes such as permanent injury or death. In many cases risk management is primarily concerned with damage control; that is, activities to reduce the likelihood of litigation. Risk management can also have a positive side when it generates activities to prevent error and adverse events. This chapter addresses the basis for such activities.

A simple heuristic method of addressing the question of why an error occurs is presented in this chapter. Prior to describing that method, the reasons for the importance of identifying such factors is addressed. These reasons include the harm that adverse events cause, the cost of such events, the prevailing attitude toward error and the implications of that attitude for determining why incidents occur. After the method is discussed, examples of its applications to actual incidents are described. Implications are presented for the use of the method in identifying factors that contribute to near misses and potential incidents, as well as reducing the likelihood of events with adverse outcomes. Lastly, the importance of searching for why errors occur is discussed in terms of enhancing the effectiveness of healthcare, patient safety and quality of life.

ERRORS AND ADVERSE EVENTS

Examples of Adverse Events:

Errors in healthcare are manifest in a variety of ways: an elderly resident in a nursing home nearly strangles in bed, an infant in a neonatal intensive care unit is burned by a pulse oximeter, a surgical patient is unresponsive because of receiving too much morphine, a child being monitored for a heart condition is electrocuted, a diabetic has an adverse reaction from insulin mis-management. In each of those examples, error is inferred from an event. Most often error is considered as resulting from an adverse event (AE) linked to an adverse outcome of death or serious injury.

Error can also be manifest in an incident with no clinically significant adverse outcome or an incident that was aborted before an adverse outcome occurred. Examples of such almost adverse events (AAEs) are: inappropriate programming of an infusion pump (the computer chip-based device that regulates the drip rate of a solution or medication into a patient) though the amount of drug administered was so low that there was no apparent adverse outcome; a clinician realised that a wrong drug had been drawn from a vial and the injection was aborted at the last minute; a surgical electro-cautery device with a hot tip was being placed on a flammable patient drape by a surgeon - when a nurse spoke a warning the device was removed.

A third class of errors are those that are waiting to happen, potential adverse events (PAEs). Examples of PAEs are anything used in healthcare that requires extra attention for its safe and effective operation, such as the plastic plunger holder that doesn't fit the plunger in a syringe pump (an infusion pump that has a drug filled syringe attached with the plunger in a plastic holder to push the appropriate amount of drug into the solution); no feedback in programmable devices; vials that look alike but contain very different drugs; warning alarms that do not indicate the cause of the alarm.

Cost of Error

There are costs of AEs in terms of suffering and loss of life; and there also are financial costs. The magnitude of the financial costs of error exclusive of litigation is staggering. Information from a large, carefully controlled study of preventable AEs in hospitalised patients during one calendar year (Leape *et al.*, 1991) extrapolated for the entire country provides the basis for estimating dollar cost. That cost, which includes medical treatment for the AEs, deaths, lost wages and lost household production, but no consideration of pain and suffering or legal fees, was estimated to be $25 billion (Bogner, 1994). That is the cost only for AEs judged as preventable – the total cost of all AEs is considerably more. It should be noted that the information for the study was gathered in 1984 , before the introduction of managed care in the United States.

The applicability of the cost information from 15 years ago to the cost of AEs in today's healthcare is a matter for further research; however, the magnitude of the estimated cost has far-reaching implications. Savings from reducing AEs could have considerable impact on a number of social issues, including the cost of additional medical care necessitated by AEs and the cost of health insurance premiums.

A further cost of AEs is that indirectly incurred by the healthcare facility. The publicity from the well documented case of the death of Betsy Lehman, an editor of the Health Section of the Boston *Globe*, from a four-fold overdose of a very toxic chemotherapy drug at Dana Farber Medical Center in Boston was considered the cause of investors backing out of an agreement to buy bonds issued to construct a research building at the Center (Knox and Blanton, 1995). Thus, in addition to humanitarian reasons, there are fiscal incentives for the health care facility, the patients and their families and society in general to reduce the likelihood of error in healthcare. With the cost of error so great and the implications of that cost so profound, why is more not being done to address it? A major reason is the prevailing attitude toward error.

Attitudes Toward Error

The seriousness and culpability of error tends to be judged by the severity of its outcome. The cause of an error tends to be seen simply as the person who committed the error that ultimately led to the adverse outcome. This straightforward, but simplistic, view has a number of implications.

First, if it is assumed that the sole cause of an error is the person associated with it, then the only target for action to reduce the likelihood of the error recurring is that person. With the cause of the AE identified, there is no impetus to analyse the situation for error-encouraging factors. However, an error, as will be shown later, usually results from a co-occurrence of several conditions or precursor events, each of which may be necessary, but none alone is sufficient to induce the error.

Secondly, the presumption that the care provider is the sole cause of the error often results in disciplinary action and sometimes the removal of the person concerned. If conditions in the context of care predisposed the person to error (Cooper *et al.*, 1978), then removal of that person will not necessarily reduce the likelihood of error. For example, if an individual considered grossly careless in committing an AE is removed from the position and the case considered closed, the question remains as to why that person was careless. If the individual is not consistently careless, the reason must be sought elsewhere. If the individual was consistently careless in providing healthcare, the question is why were they allowed to provide care in the first place and why was action not taken sooner.

Removing the person does not address the heart of the problem. The conditions that contributed to the error remain to predispose another person to error. This is analogous to a play, with the context of care being the script. The actors may change, but the script (the conditions contributing to error) remains to influence the actors' performance. The way to change the performance (to reduce AEs) is to change the script. To do that effectively, it is necessary to identify the factors that contribute to error and target them for change. To accomplish this, it is necessary to resist the temptation to simply punish the person concerned, an action that meets the need for retribution and instead to examine the context of the AE for error-inducing factors. This approach to error does not absolve the individual of responsibility. The individual is responsible not for the act *per se* but for allowing the error-conducive conditions to exist without taking action to change them. This systems approach to medical error is well expressed by Billings (1997) in the context of a discussion of error in aviation:

"Without full information concerning the context and environment(s) in which accidents occur, it is not possible to understand their genesis and how to take rational steps to prevent future accidents. Accidents are not only human failures, they are also failures of design, operation, maintenance . . . In short they are system failures" (p. 147-48).

CONTEXT OF ERROR

Error Context as Systems

Although the term 'system' is used throughout this chapter, it is defined briefly here to provide a common frame of reference for this discussion. The term 'system' refers to a category of factors or characteristics which interacts with characteristics of other systems or categories. Although the literature is not replete with such contributing factors in healthcare, research in other domains has identified factors that constitute systems. The findings from aviation, transportation, nuclear power, the military and industry have been synthesised into categories of factors by Moray (1994), Rasmussen (1994) and Senders and Moray (1991) among others. The systems which comprise the context for health care described below are an amalgam of those categories, with an elaboration of Moray's (1994) proposition that central to the system of the context of care is a physical device, which for ease of reference in this discussion represents any means of providing care, such as medication, exercise, therapeutic procedures, or collecting information to be used in diagnosis.

This elaboration of the systems concept is based on the observation that the device does not operate in isolation; a user or care provider and care recipient must be involved. For all those involved in the provision of care, the context includes the ambient conditions, physical setting, social situation, organisational culture and expectations, and legal-regulatory proscriptions and cultural mores. These systems function as concentric circles, with the influence of each circle affecting those within its circumference and all impacting on the entities of the care-providing nucleus. Examples of characteristics of each system are represented in Table 5.1.

TABLE 5.1

System characteristics that contribute to medical error.

	Examples of characteristics
Legal-Regulatory-Cultural	Litigation fears, regulatory concerns, reimbursement, national culture.
Organisation	Workload, hours worked, reports, policies for caring for uninsured, organisational culture.
Social	Other care providers, family members, professional culture.
Physical	Placement of medical devices, room size, furniture, availability of electricity, water.
Ambient	Altitude, illumination, temperature, noise.

Care providing:
    Provider
 	
    Device
    Patient
	
	Knowledge, skills, target task experience, stamina.
	For home care: age, health status.
	Purpose, moveable or mounted, technological sophistication.
	Presenting problem, age, body weight, co-morbidity, anxiety.

Authors of a study of adverse drug events concluded that a systems approach is a viable way to address error (Leape *et al.*, 1995). The systems approach in that study, of individual chart review and personal interviews, is quite labour intensive and so is not amenable to adoption on a large scale. To be practically viable, it is necessary that the systems approach can be easily applied to identify factors that contribute to error in individual events. The method discussed in the next section addresses this issue.

METHOD FOR IDENTIFYING THE WHY OF ERROR

Assessment Methodology

The assessment methodology for the systems approach to medical error is based on the presumption that practicing healthcare providers are the best sources of information about factors in their own environment which may contribute to error. Self-reported free text has been considered by many, including the aviation industry (Reynard *et al.*, 1986), as the most viable way to obtain comprehensive information about an event. A totally open, free response methodology, however, allows for the perpetuation of common presumptions, particularly the tendency to blame people for errors involving human activity. This is especially the case for healthcare professionals, who assume responsibility for error as their professional obligation; they may blame themselves even though the error involved a device or procedure that was nearly impossible to use.

Respondents also may only consider factors in their immediate environment without considering the impact of other, system, factors. For example, selecting drug A when seeking drug B could be attributed to lack of attention by the healthcare provider. In this example, cues to systems factors could prompt a report that the drug containers were unexpectedly different from what was typical. That response could lead to an investigation that reveals an unannounced cost-saving change in suppliers, resulting in changes in the appearance of the containers.

The Systems Approach Assessment Tool

The assessment tool is a variation of the Critical Incident Technique (CIT) (Flanagan, 1954). The CIT has been modified by a number of clinicians and researchers when considering anesthesia incidents. Short *et al.* (1992) developed a questionnaire based on the CIT that requested a description of the incident including associated and contributory factors, to which a care provider who witnessed the incident would respond anonymously. The systems approach assessment tool is a further modification the CIT. It reduces the structure of the questionnaire yet retains its spirit in the form of a checklist of the systems categories in Table 5.1. A checklist of these characteristics and examples which serve as memory aids, appears as Appendix A.

Care providers do not always have time to write down a detailed description of an incident and they tend to forget aspects of the incident after a period of time. Demand characteristics of an interview situation could compromise the accuracy of reporting the factors in an incident. With the checklist, care providers can quickly make notes by category at the time of the incident; those notes will be a reminder when they have time to record additional information. As information is gathered and analysed, the findings guide refinements of the checklist, such as sub-sections of factors in specific systems or for individual services.

Requesting checklists for AAEs and PAEs not only provides information to avert AEs, it can also increase the incidence of reporting. Some may consider an AAE as always indicating culpability, interpreting it as incompetence thwarted by good fortune; a PAE, however, which describes a condition, situation, or set of factors perceived as an error waiting to happen, is a constructive, safety conscious, preventive activity. Because of the nature of the assessment tool, analysis of information obtained from it can provide insights into error-prone conditions that transcend the specific incidents.

ANALYSES OF CASE EXAMPLES

Elements of the description of an incident obtained from the systems checklist can be arrayed as an analysis matrix. Elements in the matrices can be compared to determine consistencies of factors across events involving the same device, across events for a given system characteristic, such as the work shift on which events occur, or across a population with a common third party payer. The following examples of the systems approach to analysis of error are elaborations of examples described at the beginning of this chapter.

The first example concerns an elderly person nearly strangled in a hospital bed. A nurse walking by a patient's room in the middle of the night heard an unusual sound. When the lights were turned on, the nurse saw that the patient had her head between the bedside rails and her body was wedged between the mattress and bed frame. The patient clearly was in distress; the nurse intervened and there was no apparent injury. The nurse provided systems information, which is presented in Table 5.2.

A number of factors in several systems contributed to this AAE. Among those factors was the diminutive size of the patient with respect to the size of the gap between the mattress and bedframe and the time the incident was discovered, a time when staff activity is at its lowest. Information from this analysis, together with information from similar incidents, can be persuasive in advocating increased checking on frail elderly patients during the night and modification of bedframe-mattress gaps, as well as alerting the purchasing department to the importance of checking equipment for the possibility of entrapment.

TABLE 5.2

Analysis Matrix for Example 1

Analysis Matrix for	AE ___
Actual AEs, Almost AEs (AAE), and Potential AEs (PAEs)	AAE x
	PAE ___

Event: Patient head caught in bed side rails; body wedged between bed frame & mattress
Time: 4 a.m. Sunday
Location: Patient's room in 200 bed community hospital

System or Context	Characteristics
Legal-regulatory-cultural	Managed care, very sick patients
Organisation	Heavy workload, vague treatment protocols
Social	Hysterical daughter afraid mother will die
Physical	Semi-private room, 2 monitors, 2 infusion pumps – 1 apparently stored in room
Ambient	Light off and heat high by daughter's request
Care provider	Contract nurse, 2nd consecutive 12 hr shift, feels catching flu
Means of providing care	Bed side rails have 10 inch opening between 2 horizontal, 2 bar sections, mattress not flush with bed frame
Patient	84 year old, 95 pound woman, with diabetes and pneumonia

Example 2: A Neonate at Risk from a Monitor

The second example concerns an infant in a Neonatal Intensive Care Unit (NICU) who was burned by a pulse oximeter, a device with a heat producing sensor that provides information about the oxygen concentration in the blood. Typically, the oximeter is placed on a finger or taped to the skin. Because the hand size and activity of a neonate makes a finger placement impractical, the device is taped to the infant's skin, often the leg. The heat of the sensor can burn an infant's delicate skin if the device is not moved to a new site every 3 hours. The nurse's aide provided the system information that is arrayed in the analysis matrix in Table 5.3.

TABLE 5.3

Analysis Matrix for Example 2

Analysis Matrix for	AE _x_
Actual AEs, Almost AEs (AAE), and Potential AEs (PAEs)	AAE___
	PAE___

Event: Severe burn of right leg.

Time: 3 a.m. Sunday

Location: Patient's bassinette in 10 patient Neonatal Intensive Care Unit (NICU) in 200 bed community hospital

---

System or Context	Characteristics
Legal-regulatory-cultural	Managed care patient, child of immigrant parents from the Middle-East
Organisation	NICU at capacity with 10 very critical patients
Social	Registered Nurse (RN) uncommunicative to aide, unavailable.
Physical	Open area. All patients have multiple monitors
Ambient	Lighted area, multiple alarms sounding, some infants crying
Care provider	Aide only person in NICU, 2nd consecutive 12 hour shift, 3 months in NICU, first night with the specific RN. Contract RN first night on NICU, 2nd consecutive 12 hr shift, also assigned to sparsely occupied adjacent Cardiac Intensive Care Unit (CICU)
Means of providing care	Pulse oximeter alarms only when oxygen concentration drops below a designated level
Patient	3 day old, 5 pound male infant with congenital heart defects, intubated (tube inserted in trachea for ventilator assisted breathing), burn where oximeter was taped. Both parents have red hair

---

The analysis suggests that the workload for the aide is excessive in terms of the number and condition of the NICU patients, the skills required to treat the patients and the availability of assistance from the registered nurse (RN). Because the aide's vigilance was being compromised by excessive demands, coupled with the lack of alarm or other signal to indicate when to move the device, the device was not moved as prescribed. The infant's skin was particularly sensitive due to inherited coloration. Because of intubation, the infant could not cry to indicate pain from the burn; the level of ambient noise probably masked the attention-getting sound of any excessive movement by the patient.

Information from the analysis provides the basis for several activities: review and revision of staffing assignments, the installation of a signal that can be identified over the ambient noise to indicate when to move the device and an interview with the RN to discuss the lack of communication. In the interview the RN reported that she was in pain from a recent root canal operation and that the patients in the CICU needed more attention than anticipated, which underscored the need to revise staffing.

The value of the analysis matrix in identifying factors that contribute to incidents in a facility becomes apparent when matrices are inspected for consistencies across settings in a given healthcare facility. Such a consistency is evident when comparing the matrices for examples 1 and 2: both incidents occurred around 4 a.m. This presents a persuasive argument to examine the viability of the night shift staffing. If management did not address the problems, information from the analysis matrices could deflect the attribution of responsibility for an incident from an individual to the system that did not respond to an identified problem.

Example 3: Excessive Dose of Morphine

A third example is of a patient found by the nurse in an unresponsive condition after receiving a 50 mg bolus of morphine from an infusion pump. The administration tubing was found to be inserted incorrectly into the pump, which resulted in an over-delivery of morphine (Brown *et al.*, 1997). Information concerning this AE was obtained from Freedom of Information Act Releaseable Medical Device Reports submitted to the US Food and Drug Administration, coupled with site visits to a hospital's surgical floor. The systems approach to that information is represented by the analysis matrix in Table 5.4.

TABLE 5.4

Analysis Matrix for Example 3

<table>
<tr><td colspan="2" align="center">Analysis Matrix for
Actual AEs, Almost AEs (AAE), and Potential AEs (PAEs)</td><td>AE __
AAE x
PAE__</td></tr>
</table>

Event: Patient unresponsive
Time: 8 p.m. Wednesday
Location: Surgical floor in 500 bed for-profit hospital

System or Context	Characteristics
Legal-regulatory-cultural	Managed care patient, hospital due for accreditation review
Organisation	Floor full to capacity with patients recovering from major surgery
Social	Husband and son at bedside, both continually asking questions
Physical	Semi-private room with second bed empty. Patients had multiple monitors
Ambient	Light dimmed at patient's request. Television program with sound in progress
Care provider	Nurse's aide primary care giver. First time the aide worked on surgical service. Prior to reporting for work, the aide worked a 12 hour shift at a local nursing home. One RN available on the floor
Means of providing care	Infusion pump had similar appearance to others in use on the floor. Pump in this AAE is loaded starting at the bottom of the pump; others are loaded from the top. Instructions for different loading are provided on inside of door near hinges in small font with some drawing in a small format
Patient	67 year old Caucasian female, 2 days post knee replacement surgery in considerable pain. Patient experienced no apparent negative consequences from the incident

There are no warnings or other indications of incorrect tubing insertion on the infusion pump, so the aide was not alerted to a problem. There is no fail-safe component that would physically preclude incorrect insertion of tubing into the pump. Because the pump looked like pumps that are loaded differently, it was loaded in the more familiar manner, which allowed free-flow of the drug. The dim light and angle of view made it difficult to see a problem in the drip chamber; the ambient noise was distracting.

Information from this analysis could be used to advocate removal of that model infusion pump from use, alert purchasing to the need for safety features in future pump purchases, and inform the manufacturer of the problem. If fiscal constraints preclude removing the pump from service, the information could be used to encourage marking the bottom loading pumps, perhaps by bright orange tape, to alert the user of the different manner of loading.

Example 4: The Electrocution of a Young Girl

The fourth example is of a 4 year old girl who was electrocuted. She was being treated for a number of birth defects, which involved the use of multiple medical devices. In searching for the cord for the heart monitor to connect to the lead from the electrodes taped to the child's chest, the nurse found a cord that fitted the pin configuration on the lead. The cord was presumed to belong to the heart monitor, when in fact it was detached from an infusion pump which was running on battery, but still connected to the electrical outlet. When the cord was connected to the lead, the power surged through the electrodes to the child's heart. Basic information for the analysis matrix presented as Table 5.5 was obtained from a case study of the incident (Casey, 1998).

The systems approach analysis to this AE identified factors in the physical environment that contributed to error, such as the proximity of the infusion pump and its cord to the heart monitor. Analysis of both the involved devices points to the lack of information provided by devices; the power cord for the infusion pump should be clearly identifiable as being a power cord and the heart monitor cord should be clearly identifiable and different fittings for the two cords should preclude such mis-connections. Information from this analysis could be used to modify the equipment by painting color coding on power cords and devices and to inform purchasing to be aware of the need for physical failsafe mechanisms when buying equipment.

TABLE 5.5
Analysis Matrix for Example 4

Analysis Matrix for Actual AEs, Almost AEs (AAE), and Potential Aes (PAEs)	AE __x__ AAE___ PAE ___

Event: Death by electrocution.
Time: 10 a.m. Tuesday
Location: Patient's bed in a chronic care facility.

System or Context	Characteristics
Legal-regulatory-cultural	Managed care patient, concern for fiscal obligation for care of a patient who would always need extensive care.
Organisation	Chronic care facility near full capacity.
Social	Immigrant father and 2 restless brothers age 6 months and 2 years at bedside.
Physical	Area crowded with equipment and stuffed animals.
Ambient	Lit area, brothers noisy, father yelling at sons.
Care provider	Contract nurse, only other time at facility was 5 months earlier.
Means of providing care	Bedside area crowded with devices. Tangle of cables, cords, and tubes. No color or tactile coding of cable or leads. No obvious indication that infusion pump is running on battery.
Patient	4 year old female, multiple birth defects, low weight, unresponsive.

Example 5: A Diabetic with Inappropriate Insulin Dosage

The final example concerns a diabetic patient who presented with problems from inappropriate insulin dosage at an Emergency Room (ER) in Denver, Colorado. The patient tested her blood sugar with a blood glucose meter (BGM), a computer chip based device that senses the glucose level in blood placed on a strip inserted into the device. Adjustments to insulin dosage, diet, and exercise are based on numbers indicating the glucose level displayed on the BGM. Information provided by an emergency medical technician (EMT) appears in the analysis matrix in Table 5.6.

TABLE 5.6

Analysis Matrix for Example 5

Analysis Matrix for Actual AEs, Almost AEs (AAE), and Potential AEs (PAEs)	AE ___ AAE _x_ PAE___

Event: Diabetic coma.
Time: 2 p.m. Sunday
Location: Patient's home in Denver, CO.

System or Context	Characteristics
Legal-regulatory-cultural	Medicare patient recent Hispanic immigrant.
Organisation	Ambulance to ER of city hospital.
Social	Distraught elderly sister and brother accompanied patient. Neither EMT nor ambulance driver knew Spanish. Additional family members came to ER; only one could speak rudimentary English..
Physical	Ambulance crowded with relatives. Access to patient difficult. No appropriate family waiting area in ER.
Ambient	Noise from concerned family. Light obstructed by family members. Altitude.
Care provider	Experienced. No knowledge of Spanish by any available personnel.
Means of providing care	Use of BGM reviewed with patient and family.
Patient	70 year old non-English speaking Hispanic female, insulin dependent diabetic for 40 years, overweight. Successfully brought out of coma.

At first consideration, this AE could seem to be user error; however, the systems approach analysis identified a factor in a context system, an ambient condition that compromises the accuracy of BGM readings – altitude. Denver is the 'mile high' city and altitude affects the chemical reaction of the BGM test strips. That can produce an inaccurate reading, which leads to inappropriate management of the disease. No amount of user training would correct a presumed error using the BGM. It is not a user error but a problem with the device under the high altitude conditions. Information from this analysis can be provided by Diabetic Nurse Educators and physicians so they can alert their patients to the problem, develop short-term ways to avoid AEs based on inaccurate BGM readings and bring the problem to the attention of the manufacturers and insist on correction.

Viability of the Systems Approach

Although the systems approach checklist was developed to assist in gathering incident information, its variant, the analysis matrix, can be used to array information from published sources as illustrated in examples 3 and 4 as well as information gathered by individuals involved in or witnessing an incident. When the information is not gathered using the checklist, some extrapolation, user consultation, or site visitation may be necessary to identify system factors.

Arraying information by systems also can make salient otherwise obscured factors that contribute to incidents, such as altitude in example 5. Information from an analysis matrix could also indicate incipient problems which otherwise might go unnoticed, such as the lack of Spanish speaking emergency personnel in example 5. Comparison of matrices across incidents can identify common problems, such as the night shift staffing in examples 1 and 2. Although the systems approach checklist and analysis matrix are not techniques amenable to statistical analysis, they are potent means of identifying patterns of factors which contribute to error and reveal commonalities across incidents, thus providing insights into the etiology of incidents, the 'why' of error.

THE BENEFITS OF A SYSTEMS APPROACH TO HEALTHCARE

The systems approach expands the consideration of the cause of error beyond the individual or individuals associated with the event to factors in the context of systems in which the event occurred and provides documentation of the influence of factors that contribute to error. Information identifying error-encouraging system factors that is obtained from the systems checklist and analysis matrix can be used to substantiate problems and institute efforts for change to reduce the likelihood of error. Rather than addressing a symptom of a problem, the person associated with an error, the systems approach identifies aspects of the problem which, when addressed, will reduce recurrence of the symptoms. Thus, when a healthcare provider whose cognitive capabilities are compromised by stress and fatigue from excessive workload in a managed care setting is involved in an error, the systems approach analysis provides documented information on contributing factors such as reimbursement policies to support arguments to address and revise the factors. Similarly, if health care facility procedures are found to contribute to AEs, AAEs, and PAEs, those findings provide documented support for change that cannot be dismissed as complaints from disgruntled staff.

The approach described can be used easily in any setting. This is important because of the variety of contexts in which care is provided: in the home, in the playground, in camp, at shopping centres, in sports arena, on the battlefield – in short, anywhere people gather. Care is provided in many forms, to widely differing groups of people in often rapidly changing conditions. Probably no other domain has as many systems conditions that affect task performance, or conditions that vary so precipitously – conditions that induce error.

The systems approach also enhances the sensitivity of care providers to error inducing factors. The checklist and analysis matrix are easy to use. They involve no extensive instructions or training. Rather, as stated at the outset of this chapter, those tools comprise a simple, heuristic method for identifying factors that contribute to error and AEs, AAEs and PAEs. Those who describe incidents can become involved in the detective-like search for factors that contribute to error by comparing factors arrayed in an analysis matrix across events in the same or diverse settings in any way that may be useful for the purpose at hand or to satisfy curiosity. They can be heartened by the strong basis for action afforded by consistencies in factors associated with error. It is understandable that management, industry, or society is resistant to change when only verbal complaints are presented. Documented information that identifies factors that contribute to error is more likely to be accepted. The solicitation of descriptions of PAEs is an important goal. There is no possible culpability in reporting potential incidents, so care providers can describe them without fear of litigation or reprisal. This could be a step on the road to considering error as a gem, something to be treasured because it provides information that can lead to improvement.

In summary, the systems approach reflects the quest for understanding in actual, almost, or potential adverse events or errors in health care. It is a viable and potent tool for the management of such factors to effectively reduce the likelihood of adverse outcomes associated with error or to avoid incidents. The incorporation of the systems approach throughout health care can effectively reduce the likelihood of error and prevent identified potential adverse events from becoming actual. The systems approach to adverse events can benefit healthcare by moderating risk, enhancing safety and reducing the human and fiscal impact of error.

REFERENCES

Billings, C. E. (1997). *Aviation Automation: The Search for a Human-Centered Approach.* Lawrence Erlbaum Associates, Mahwah, NJ.

Bogner, M. S. (1994). Human error in medicine: A frontier for change. In: *Human Error in Medicine* (M. S. Bogner, ed.), pp. 373-383, Lawrence Erlbaum Associates, Mahwah, NJ.

Brown, S. L., M. S., Bogner, C. M. Parmentier and J. B. Taylore (1997). Human error and patient-controlled analgesia pumps. *Journal of Intravenous Nursing,* **20**, 311-317.

Casey, S.M. (1998). *Set Phasers on Stun.* Aegean Publishing Company, Santa Barbara, CA.

Cooper, J. B., R. C. Newbower, C. D. Long and B. McPeek (1978). Preventable anesthesia mishaps: A study of human factors. *Anesthesiology,* **49**, 399-406.

Flanagan, J. C. (1954). The critical incident technique. *Psychological Bulletin,* **51**, 327-358.

Knox, R. A. and K. Blanton (1995). Overdoses cloud Dana-Farber bonds. Boston *Globe,* Economy Section, p. 77, March 24.

Leape, L. L., T. A. Brennan, N. Laird, A. G. Lawthers, A. R. Localio, B. A Barnes, L. Herbert, J. O. Newhouse, P. C. Weiler and H. Hiatt (1991). The nature of adverse events in hospitalized patients. *New England Journal of Medicine,* **324**, 377-384.

Leape, L. L., D. W. Bates, D. J. Culllen, J. Cooper, , H. J. Demonaco, T. Gallivan, R. Hallisay, J. Ives, N. Laird, G. Laffel, R. Nemeski, L. A. Peterson, J. Porter, D. Serv, B. F. Shea S. D. Small, B. J. Sweitzer, T. Thompson and M. Vander Viet (1995). Systems analysis of adverse drug events. *Journal of the American Medical Association,* **274**, 35-43.

Moray, N. (1994). Error reduction as a systems problem. In: *Human Error in Medicine* (M. S. Bogner, ed.), pp. 67-91, Lawrence Erlbaum Associates, Inc, Mahwah, NJ.

Rasmussen, J. (1994). Afterword. In: *Human Error in Medicine* (M.S. Bogner, ed.), pp. 385-394, Lawrence Erlbaum Associates, Inc, Mahwah, NJ.

Reynard, W. D., C. E., Billings, E. S. Cheaney and R. Hardy (1986). NASA Reference Publication 1114 *The Development of the NASA Aviation Safety Reporting System.* Washington, DC: National Aeronautics and Space Administration Scientific and Technical Information Branch.

Senders, J. W. and N. P. Moray (1991). *Human Error: Cause, Prediction, and Reduction.* Lawrence Erlbaum Associates, Inc, Mahwah, NJ.

Short, T. G., A. O'Regan, J. Lew and T.E. Oh (1992). Critical incident reporting in an anaesthetic department quality assurance programme. *Anesthesia,* **47**, 3-7.

APPENDIX A

Checklist with Examples as Memory Aids*

AE ___
AAE__
PAE__

Incident:
Time:
Location:

System or Context	Factors
Legal-regulatory-cultural	*litigation fears, regulatory concerns, reimbursement, national values
Organisation	*workload, staff support, hours worked, reports, policies, organizational culture
Social	*other care providers, family members, professional culture
Physical	*placement of medical devices, room size, furniture, space for charting
Ambient	*illumination, temperature, noise, altitude
Care provider	* knowledge, skills, target task experience, stamina
Means of providing care: devices, drugs, information for diagnosis	*ease of use of device, technological sophistication, clarity of medication labels, procedures, clarity of lab reports, packaging
Patient	*presenting problem, age, weight, co-morbidity, anxiety, allergies

*Examples can be customized with examples pertinent to specific setting or omitted as desired.

Chapter 6

Clinical Accident Analysis: Understanding the Interactions Between the Task, Individual, Team and Organisation

Sally Taylor-Adams*, Charles Vincent, Clinical Risk Unit, Department of Psychology, University College London, UK

*HRRI Lecturer in Clinical Risk

Introduction

Hospital adverse patient outcomes are frequent (Leape, 1994) and the risk of iatrogenic injury to patients in acute hospitals remains high, with studies reporting between 4% and 17% of patients sustaining injury (Mills, 1995; Brennan *et al.*, 1991; Wilson, 1995 and Andrews, 1997). The cost of such incidents is increasing at an alarming rate: the department of health has calculated that more than £200 million will be spent on clinical adverse event claims in the year 2000, in the UK. The cost of individual accidents can be large - for example, the settlement for a child left permanently physically and mentally handicapped following birth trauma can regularly exceed £1.5 million. The payment of such large sums of money not only has the potential to destabilise trusts, it also eats into trust budgets, which may prevent other services being provided to patients. Even with the advent of clinical audit, comparatively few studies in medicine focus directly on the causes of adverse events, with some notable exceptions such as the confidential enquiries into maternal and perioperative deaths (Buck *et al.*, 1987; HMSO, 1994). Leape (1994) has argued that if we are to understand adverse events, more attention must be given to psychological and human factors research on the nature, mechanisms and causes of errors, particularly the fact that liability of error is strongly affected by the context and conditions of work. Critical incident and organisational analyses of individual cases have illustrated the complexity of the chain of events that may lead to an adverse outcome (Cooper *et al.*, 1984; Cook *et al.*, 1994). The root causes of an adverse event may lie in a variety of interlocking factors, such as the use of locums, communication and supervision problems, excessive workload and so on. Some fundamental features of a unit, such as communication within a team, may be implicated in a wide variety of adverse clinical events (Vincent, 1997).

The systematic analysis of accidents and serious incidents is a fundamental feature of most industrial safety programmes. Current approaches to safety in medicine are very different from those in industry. Safety management in medicine tends to focus on retrospective case analysis where a large number of cases are reviewed and blame is attributed to the staff rather than identifying the underlying system failures and little seems to be done to reduce error in the future. Occurrence screening, medical audit and the analysis of closed claims tend to be the approaches adopted by medics to investigate error. Until recently there have been few entry points for human factors specialists. However, the field is developing rapidly in healthcare and the case for human factors approaches is becoming clearer. Clinical risk management offers a possible avenue for human factors specialists, as it is an approach to quality and safety which specifically targets adverse events and is modelled on risk management approaches in other settings.

It is currently the case in UK hospitals that serious incidents may be discussed with colleagues or in departmental audit and review meetings, but few studies or reports of such meetings are published, making it difficult to develop a systematic method of investigation. Incidents that may lead to litigation are investigated intensively, with the focus on whether care was substandard and whether it caused identifiable injury. However, investigations are often undertaken years after the event, when litigation is brought, and analyses rely on the medical records, which may be missing, incomplete and which in any case cannot give a complete account of the actions of the staff involved. Furthermore, lawyers are seldom interested in why care was sub-standard, so factors such as staff members being undertrained, exhausted or inadequately supervised are rarely considered. Incident reporting and analysis will hopefully improve this lamentable state of affairs.

The Development of Human Factors Approaches in Medicine

The assessment of accidents in large scale socio-technical systems has a high profile in industry, after such disasters as Bhopal, Chernobyl and Piper Alpha. The human factors community has developed a variety of methods of analysis, which have begun to be adapted for use in medical contexts (Bogner, 1994). This has led to a much broader understanding of accident causation, with less focus on the individual who makes an error and more on pre-existing organisational factors that provide the conditions in which errors occur (Reason, 1995). Reason has also suggested that the results of such investigations "have clearly shown that medical mishaps share many important causal similarities with the breakdown of complex socio-technical systems". If the lessons learnt in one industry can be transferred to another, the effort and energy required to solve system safety problems will be greatly enhanced. The oil, chemical and nuclear industries have developed tools to systematically analyse organisational safety performance (Wagenaar *et al.*, 1994; Hurst *et al.*, 1994; Johnson, 1980). These approaches assess safety qualitatively via the presence or absence of safety indicators. Typically there is a general framework, with industry specific components.

Reason's (1993, 1995) model was originally developed for use in complex industrial systems as a mechanism for understanding the causes of serious accidents and to identify methods of accident prevention. We have used it to analyse more than twenty cases in obstetrics and mental health (Stanhope *et al.*, 1997; Taylor-Adams *et al.*, 1999), and have adapted it considerably in the process. The method is essentially to examine the chain of events that leads to an accident or an adverse event, consider the actions of those involved and then, crucially, to look further back at the conditions in which staff were working and the organisational context in which the incident occurred. This model has been explained in detail in Carthey *et al.'s* chapter (chapter 7). The first step in any analysis is to identify the active failures - unsafe acts or omissions committed by those at the 'sharp-end' of the system (pilots, anaesthetists, nurses, etc) whose actions can have immediate adverse consequences. To translate this model into the medical domain we have re-named active failures 'clinical management problems' (CMPs). For each identified CMP the assessor is required to record the salient clinical events at that time (e.g. bleeding heavily, blood pressure falling, etc.) and other patient factors affecting the process of care (e.g. patient very distressed, etc) so as to give a medical context to the adverse event. Having identified the active failures (CMPs) the analysis then considers the conditions in which errors occur and the wider organisational context. These factors include such factors as high workload and fatigue; inadequate knowledge, ability or experience; a stressful environment; rapid organisational change, etc. These are the factors which influence staff performance and which may precipitate error and affect patient outcomes.

A Framework for the Analysis of Risk in Medicine

The framework described below was initially based on Reason's model. However, we have extended and adapted this model substantially for use in a medical context. Principally we have produced a series of taxonomies classifying the error producing conditions (contributory factors) in a single framework, which can affect clinical practice (Vincent *et al.*, 1998).

The framework is summarised in Table 6.1. To ensure that the framework is comprehensive and mutually exclusive, we have reviewed the major frameworks in use in the human factors field, such as the socio-technical pyramid of Hurst and Ratcliff (1994), taxonomies contained within human reliability quantification tools, such as HEART (Williams, 1986) and THERP (Swain and Guttmann, 1983), to ensure that all factors of potential relevance to medicine were included. In addition to a review of the human factors literature, the human factors researcher (ST-A) spent a considerable amount of time within hospitals observing care pathways and recording information on factors specific to medicine that can influence performance, e.g. the staff-patient relationship.

At the bottom, in the sense of being the most direct influence on practice and outcome, are patient factors. Clearly the condition from which the patient suffers is the most powerful direct predictor of actual outcome. However, the patient's condition may also influence the quality of care in that adverse events are more likely when the patient is already seriously ill (Brennan, 1991; Giraud, 1993). Other factors, such as the patient's language and personality, may also influence communication with staff and in turn the likelihood of an adverse event. A number of staff factors, such as personality, experience and training may be influential. The confidence and assurance of staff may be of considerable importance, especially where junior staff are concerned; risk is attached to being nervous and unsure, but also to being over-confident and arrogantly self-assured.

Higher up in the framework are individual (staff) factors and team factors. The knowledge, skills and experience of staff members will affect clinical practice and how an incident is dealt with. In addition, each staff member is part of a team within the inpatient or community unit and is part of the wider organisation of the hospital. The way in which an individual practices, and their impact on the patient, is constrained and influenced by other members of the team and the way they communicate, support and supervise each other. The team is influenced in turn by management actions and by decisions made at a higher level in the organisation. These include policies regarding the use of locum or agency staff, education, training and supervision and the availability of equipment and supplies. The organisation itself is affected by the institutional context, including financial constraints, external regulatory bodies and the broader economic and political climate.

TABLE 6.1

Factors Influencing Clinical Practice

FACTOR TYPES	CONTRIBUTORY FACTORS
Institutional Context	• Government policy • Macro-economic factors • National Health Service executive • Clinical Negligence Scheme for Trusts • Accreditation of trusts and staff • Regulation (General Medical Council etc) • State of knowledge in the industry • Market
1. Organisational and Management Factors	• Organisational structure • Financial resources & constraints • Policy standards and goals • Links with external organisations • Safety culture • Risks imported/exported
2. Situational Factors	• Staffing levels & skills mix • Education and training • Workload/hours of work • Environment • Availability and maintenance of equipment & supplies • Building & design • Administrative support • Movement of patients between sites • Time factors (e.g. delays) • Atmosphere
3. Team Factors	• Verbal communication between staff • Written communication • Supervision and seeking help • Congruence/consistency of aims • Leadership & responsibility • Staff/colleagues response to incidents
4. Individual (Staff) Factors	• Knowledge & Skills • Competence • Mental and physical stressors
5. Task Factors	• Task design and clarity of structure • Availability & use of protocols • Availability & accuracy of test results • Decision-making aids
6. Patient Specific Factors	• Condition (complexity & seriousness) • Treatment • Staff-patient relationship • Personal • History

Each of these levels of analysis can be expanded to provide a more detailed specification of the components of each of the major factors. From this, a finer grained specification can be derived which might consist of specific questions on each topic, which together would make up a risk assessment instrument for this particular aspect of the framework and analysis of individual incidents for the whole gamut of potential causal influences on adverse outcomes.

The framework provides a conceptual basis for analysing adverse incidents as it examines both the clinical factors and, at the higher level, organisational factors that maybe influential. It provides a method of considering not only the actions of those involved in the events surrounding the incident, but also the conditions in which staff are working and the organisational context in which the incident occurred. In doing so, it allows the whole range of possible influences to be considered and can therefore be used to guide the investigation and analysis of the incident. Further explanation of this framework can be found in Vincent *et al.* (1998).

The Medical Discipline of Obstetrics

Obstetrics is the branch of medicine concerned with childbirth and the treatment of women before (antenatal period) during (labour and delivery) and after (postnatal period) childbirth. Obstetrics, like the nuclear power and petrochemical industries, is a high technology system. It is a dynamic field of medicine, where situational variables can change quickly. It is reliant on a complex social hierarchy and uses a variety of technical equipment.

Obstetrics can be a high risk medical domain, where errors can lead to the death or injury of both mother and baby. The obstetric/midwifery system is composed of a variety of team members, all featuring different fields of expertise. These team members can be called upon at any point during pregnancy and childbirth, yet it is important that decisions and actions are communicated effectively to ensure a co-ordinated and timely delivery of care. Obstetrics, unlike many other fields of medicine, integrates the services of primary (general practitioners and community based midwives) and secondary (obstetricians, midwives, anaesthetists and paediatricians) healthcare professionals.

A midwife is a specialist in childbirth, qualified to take responsibility for women before, during and after childbirth. She has specific skills to support and understand women, she will know when to call for obstetric advice and assistance. The midwife is able to deal with all aspects of normal childbirth. An obstetrician is a doctor who specialises in medical problems to do with pregnancy and childbirth. Most routine care is provided by junior doctors (grades such as senior house officer and registrar) working along consultant obstetricians and midwives in the obstetric team. A General Practitioner (GP) is a physician who has general medical training, but has not specialised in any particular medical field. A GP is able to provide general care for all illnesses and healthcare issues. A paediatrician is a doctor specialising in the care of babies and children. The paediatrician will be present when the baby is born, if a difficult delivery is anticipated, or a problem with the baby is expected. An anaesthetist is a doctor who has specialised in the provision of pain relief during medical procedures.

In the UK, care of pregnant women antenatally is generally undertaken by community midwives and GPs. Childbirth generally occurs within a hospital, where care is provided by midwives if the delivery is progressing normally. If childbirth is following a non-normal path, care will be provided by midwives and obstetricians, the more serious the problems the more senior members of the obstetric team will be involved in the care process. When a women requires pain relief during a surgical procedure, such as caesarean section, then an anaesthetist who is trained in providing pain relief to pregnant women will be available. If the delivery is problematic or the midwife/obstetrician believes the health of the baby is compromised, then a paediatrician will also be present at the birth of the baby. Childbirth can also occur at a woman's home, and if this is the case, care will be provided by the community midwives and occasionally the GP too. If the labour/delivery begins to follow a non-normal course, then the woman will be transferred to hospital, where integrated care will be provided by the community midwives, hospital midwives and the obstetricians.

The Investigation Process

The following obstetric case is representative of an ongoing research programme which aims to develop a generic structured and systematic method of investigating adverse and near miss outcomes in medicine for clinical risk managers. Adverse clinical events were reported to the research team and a list of midwifery and obstetric staff was compiled and each member of staff was interviewed within 48 hours of the incident. Confidentiality was assured and participation was voluntary.

Previous research (Stanhope *et al.*, 1997) has suggested that inspection of the notes during interviews could be distracting because they prevent some people from being able to focus on the reasons behind their behaviour and identifying relevant factors that would not ordinarily be recorded in the notes. The case notes were reviewed after the interviews to provide further clinical details and to establish the exact order of events. The information gathered from the interviews and the notes was integrated to produce a detailed description of the event.

The Interview

The length of the interview varied for each person, depending on the time they had available and on the extent of their involvement in the case. None took longer than 20-30 minutes. In the first stage staff gave a full description of the sequence of events and their part in it. Subsequent questions followed up comments made by the interviewee and aimed to determine the reasoning behind their actions (e.g. Why did you hesitate in calling the doctor?).

After the discussion of the case, each interviewee was presented with a performance influencing factors (PIF) questionnaire and asked

(i)   to indicate which, if any, of the 30 items they felt were relevant to or had been influential in the case e.g. workload, supervision and communication;

(ii)   to give details and elaborate on any items they selected and (iii) to say if and how their work had been affected by those items.

On completion of the checklist, each person was asked two further questions:

(i)   "With the benefit of hindsight, do you think anything should have been done differently?" and

(ii)   "In the light of this case, do you think any improvements could be made to the unit?"

A full description of the procedure and staff reactions to interviews is contained in Stanhope *et al.* (1997) and Taylor-Adams *et al.* (1999).

Establishing a Chronology of Events

The first step in the analysis is to produce an agreed history of events, specifying any important areas of disagreement between accounts or between the case notes and the memories of staff. To illustrate how our investigation process in association with the framework can be used to analyse clinical incidents, one obstetrics case has been summarised (see Box 6.1). The case concerns the obstetric emergency post-partum haemorrhage (PPH). A PPH is defined as bleeding of more than 500 mls from the genital tract in the first 24 hours after delivery. It usually occurs during or immediately after the third stage of labour (delivery of the placenta), Chamberlain *et al.* (1991).

BOX 6.1

Case 1: Chronology

The case concerns a healthy 23 year old mother, whom we shall call M. The risk factor associated with M was that she had a cardiac murmur. An ECHO had been performed by the cardiology department early in her antenatal care and it was suggested in her notes that a repeat ECHO was needed and antibiotic cover prior to delivery.

8.00 M was admitted from home to the labour ward (LW) with a history of contractions since 03.00 by midwife A. The obstetric registrar also reviewed M and noted that a repeat ECHO was required as was antibiotic cover for labour.

9.50 The cardiotocograph (CTG) showed some early decelerations of the fetal heart (a possible indication of fetal distress). A vaginal examination (VE) was performed by midwife A and the cervix was found to be 6cms dilated with the membranes bulging. In view of the fetal distress it was decided in conjunction with M that midwife A would artificially rupture M's membranes (ARM) to induce labour quickly and to minimise the fetal distress.

10.15 The obstetric registrar contacted the cardiology dept to determine a care plan for M and to organise a repeat ECHO. However the registrar was told that cardiology was "too busy" to provide the necessary information.

10.30 Preparations for delivery were made by midwife A, which included contacting a paediatrician to be present at the birth due to fetal bradycardia.

10.40 A spontaneous vaginal delivery (SVD) of a live male infant occurred with meconium stained liquor being present. The placenta was delivered a few minutes later, which appeared complete. Minimal blood loss occurred during the delivery and this was estimated to be approx 100mls. However, eight minutes after the delivery midwife A noticed fresh blood oozing from the vagina. The uterus appeared well contracted, so at this point midwife A explained to M that she was bleeding and that she needed to get a doctor to help. As M was a Muslim she did not want a male doctor in the delivery room. After some discussion, M finally agreed to a doctor reviewing her, but she was extremely unhappy with this decision. At this point midwife A pressed the emergency alarm bell in the delivery suite to summon help.

10.50 Midwife B (Head of labour ward (LW)) heard a delivery suite emergency bell, but no light came on at the nurses station console to identify the delivery suite and woman needing assistance. Midwife B walked down the LW corridor to identify the source of the bell by looking for an emergency red light outside a delivery suite.

No lights were on, so midwife B assumed that the bell had been pressed inadvertently and thus had been subsequently cancelled. Five minutes later the paediatrician vacated the delivery suite and informed midwife B of the problem. Midwife B called the obstetric registrar (male) to assist and both entered M's delivery suite. Both were aware that M was bleeding profusely and that midwife A was rubbing up a contraction in an attempt to get the uterus to contract and thus prevent further blood loss. The obstetric registrar conducted a VE to determine the cause of the bleed, which was diagnosed as an uncontracted uterus and a large clot was removed from the cervix. Midwife B commenced IV syntocinon and haemacel to help the uterus to contract. The total blood loss was estimated to be 900mls.

Day 2, 9.30

M complained of feeling dizzy, which is a side affect of heavy blood loss.

14.00 M's haemoglobin (Hb) was recorded as 6.8 (a low reading which would possibly require M receiving iron tablets or a blood transfusion). The SHO was contacted, but in the interim M discharged herself from hospital, due to a poor birth experience. Consequently the community midwife was made aware of M's low Hb and was asked to follow up the outcome.

Results

Table 6.2 shows **some** of the CMPs detected in this case; the specific contributory factors (SCFs) which triggered the CMPs; and the more latent organisational management and institutional context which underlie the SPFs.

Case Discussion

Serious incidents are rare events, but may cause considerable shock and a wave of procedural changes. However, hasty ad hoc corrective measures after single incidents are not likely to produce constructive changes. In other settings a broad range of accident and near miss data is collected and subjected to analysis, so that common organisational problems can be discerned. As the psychological and organisational precursors to near misses are assumed to be similar to incidents, the root unsafe features of organisations can be highlighted before a serious incident occurs. System deficiencies can be understood and changes implemented to enhance safety and reduce the probability of a real disaster. In this paper, only one obstetric case involving a post-partum haemorrhage has been analysed, (due to space constraints). However, in reality we have analysed a series of PPH cases, so that common organisational features can be revealed and scientifically justified system changes and error reduction strategies can be generated.

Analysis of table 6.2, finds that the CMPs documented in this case are quite disparate. However, when we investigate the SPFs (and subsequent general latent failures) which trigger the CMPs failures we notice a number of common themes. The PIFs centre on issues such as verbal communication difficulties both between professions and hospital departments. Equipment failures are rife on this obstetrics ward and feature not only in this specific case, but generally throughout the department. It is quite normal for beds to fail and vital pieces of equipment like CTGs (which monitor the baby's heartbeat) to be out of order. Staff rarely report equipment malfunctions and this could be due to a variety of reasons. Firstly, because their previous experiences indicate that either nobody is available to fix the problem, or, financial resources are so strained that the department cannot afford to get the equipment fault rectified quickly. Secondly, when a piece of equipment is formally taken out of service the unit is not provided with a back-up source of equipment and therefore the unit has to work with a depleted equipment resource.

TABLE 6.2
Case Analysis Example

CASE 1

CARE MANAGEMENT PROBLEMS AND CONTRIBUTORY FACTORS

*Use one form for each of the clinical management
problems identified*

Care Management Problem

Failure to conduct cardiology ECHO and provide antibiotic cover during labour

---

Clinical Context and Patient Factors

23 year old primip in the early stages of labour presents to the LW. Patient has a cardiac mumor and requires antibiotic cover and a repeat ECHO prior to delivery, which was not done. Patient has a PPH following delivery of her infant

---

	Specific Factors	General Factors
Individual Factors	*Physical and Mental Stressors - obstetric staff motivation poor in pursuing link with cardiology dept*	
Task Factors		
Team Factors	*Verbal Communication - problems communicating between hospital depts obstetrics and cardiology* *Team Structure and Leadership - no clear definition of responsibility, in that obstetric staff did not know who was responsible for ensuring and ECHO, etc.*	*Verbal Communication - communication links between the obstetrics and cardiology dept were generally poor*
Situational Factors		

Organisational Management Factors

Policy, Standards and Goals - senior management had not developed formal channels of communication between the various hospital departments.

Safety Culture - an "us and them" culture was in operation in the trust, which facilitated a lack of support and assistance for other trust colleagues

---

Implications and Action Points

1. Review the communication channels between the obstetric and cardiologydepts in particular (but all depts in general), if inadequate generate a policy to improve communication and timely assistance when requested

2. Look at approaches to improve staff safety culture e.g..... integrated risk management practice.

This results in the staff just 'making do' and never raising the issue of equipment problems. The above case analysis shows that the following error education strategies would be advisable in this obstetric department.

1.   **Maintenance Management** - equipment malfunctions such as the alarm system not working should be rectified quickly. A formalised responsibility and communication structure needs to be developed to ensure any member of staff who encounters equipment malfunctions reports them immediately to, for example, the sister in charge of labour ward. The sister should then briefly investigate the malfunction, take the equipment out of service if necessary and then inform the maintenance department of the problem. To make the system more resistant to equipment problems, some form of redundancy should be built into the system in the form of back-up equipment if a failure occurs. At an organisational level there must be management commitment to the rectification of equipment problems, such as setting-up and maintaining maintenance contracts with contractors, so specialist equipment can be calibrated and fixed on demand. Management can also change the culture towards reporting equipment faults by instigating regular checks of equipment functionality and ensuring problems are rectified quickly.

2.   **Communication and Safety Culture** - there were a number of communication failures and supervision shortfalls in this case. For example, the cardiology and obstetrics departments had a poor working relationship and therefore when advice was sought they failed to support each other. Team building and communication skills or conflict resolution techniques could be implemented to improve team performance, communication and interaction.

3.   **Staff Competence and Motivation** - it is important that, during the training period of doctors, senior management constantly monitors staff competence and motivation, to ensure staff perform to the highest standard. It would therefore prove relevant that regular performance reviews of clinicians are undertaken by both junior and senior staff. This performance review should accompany clinicians throughout their training period, so that subsequent Trusts are aware of previous performance, competence and training needs of their staff.

4.   **Protocols** - obstetric protocols were available to help staff assist with specific medical emergencies. However, only one copy of the protocol was available on each of the obstetric wards. Obstetric protocols are generally large, unwieldy documents that are difficult to read. It would therefore prove useful if senior management could produce a summary of the protocol in the form of a filofax, so all staff could carry a personal copy with them whilst on

duty, which they can review when needed. All consultants could agree a specific treatment strategy for obstetric emergencies. The Royal College of Obstetricians and Gynaecologists, in the UK, could produce a generic obstetric protocol, which is agreed by all consultants. This would lead to standardised care and practice in obstetrics.

The analysis might suggest that the unit is riddled with unresolved problems. This is not so, and there are several features of all the cases which highlight good aspects of the unit's performance. The current analytical process focuses on a reactive approach, where all the negative aspects of individual and system failure are documented and subsequently analysed. It is therefore proposed that in addition to this rather negative review of incidents we should also identify the positive attributes, so that practitioners get a less damming picture of events and can appreciate successful individual or team performance, so that such behaviour may be replicated in subsequent cases. Some of the positive features of the case analysis are listed below.

1.   The obstetric and midwifery team co-ordinated their resources efficiently and worked well as a team in resolving the PPH.

2.   The midwives responsible for care of the woman were very responsive to her needs, which showed professionalism and commitment.

Discussion: Human Factors in Medicine

The analysis of adverse events or near misses often reveal a series of errors combined with a set of unusual circumstances which together lead to a (potentially) catastrophic outcome. This kind of approach can reveal deep rooted unsafe features of organisations that are both inefficient and potentially dangerous. Although this case did not have a serious adverse outcome, the woman discharged herself from hospital, due to a poor childbirth experience Consequently, the community midwives had to pursue this lady to ascertain if she needed any further treatment following her PPH, depleting the financial resources of the hospital. However, this case provides a considerable amount of information both about clinical matters, such as errors of judgement and a range of non-clinical contributory causes that are frequently overlooked. The benefits of analysing cases using a formal method are that it allows an analysis in a structured format based on robust psychological constructs.

This type of analysis also allows clinicians not only to identify the active failures, which they are accustomed to doing, but also the potentially more important latent failures which create the conditions in which people make errors. By providing senior clinicians and management with information on the root causes of incidents and scientifically justified error reduction strategies, they are better able to implement organisational change to prevent future problems.

The adverse event interview structure is a quick and effective methodology which can assist clinical risk managers in investigating clinical events. The PIF questionnaire performed well as a tool to encourage clinicians to think about the non-clinical factors which they felt affected their performance. It also acted as an effective prompt, jogging a person's memory about factors not mentioned in their account and as an encouragement to provide details about other issues they might otherwise have considered trivial and not worth mentioning.

There are significant advantages to investigating near misses or less severe adverse events, rather than serious incidents where litigation may ensue and there may be recrimination, feelings of guilt and shame. Near misses are less emotive and people are less likely to apportion blame. As the psychological and organisational precursors to near misses are assumed to be similar to serious incidents, the root unsafe features of organisations can be highlighted before a serious incident occurs. System deficiencies can be understood and changes implemented to enhance safety and reduce the chances of a real disaster. Further to this, error reduction strategies can be devised to prevent large scale system failure.

The review of single adverse events or a corpus of similar cases often shows that substandard care is not the fault of an individual clinician, but often due to organisational difficulties. These can manifest themselves in a variety of ways e.g. high workload, equipment difficulties, safety culture problems and communication failures. Human factors practitioners could develop organisational safety management tools, such as the complete health and safety evaluation (CHASE, Booth *et al.* (1989)) and the structured audit technique for the assessment of safety management systems (STATAS, Hurst *et al.* (1994)) as these could assist clinicians in understanding the impact of unsound organisational decisions on clinical practice.

The use of quantified risk assessments in the form of human reliability assessments would not appear to be of great relevance to healthcare systems at present, because hospitals do not have to provide safety cases as a nuclear power plant does to the nuclear installations inspectorate to prove they can operate within safe parameters. At this stage it would appear more useful to expend our energies in more qualitative assessments to help clinicians understand why quality of care can sometimes be substandard and identify ways to improve the quality of care. Research of this nature will pave the way for more systematic human factors assessments in the future.

To conclude, it appears that there are many opportunities for human factors practitioners in the healthcare system but is important that we offer useful and applicable clinical risk management tools and solutions.

REFERENCES

Andrews, L. B., C. Stocking, T. Krizek et al. (1997). An alternative strategy for studying adverse events in medical care. *Lancet*, **349**, 309-13.

Bognor, M. S. (1994). *Human Error in Medicine*. Lawrence Erlbaum, Hillsdale, New Jersey.

Booth, R.T., A.J. Boyle, A. I. Glendon, A. R. Hale and A. E. Waring (1989). CHASE II: The complete health and safety evaluation manual for the larger organisation, Version 4.1, Health and Safety Technology and Management, Birmingham.

Brennan, T. A., L. L. Leape, N. M. Laird, L. Hebert, A. R. Localio and A. G. Lawthers (1991). Incidence of adverse events and negligence in hospitalised patients: results of the Harvard medical practice study I. *New England Journal of Medicine*, **324**, 370-6.

Buck, N., H. B. Devlin and J. N. Lunn (1987). *Confidential enquiry into perioperative deaths*. London: Nuffield Provincial Hospitals Trust.

Chamberlain, G., J. Dewhurst and D. Harvey (1991). *Obstetrics Illustrated Textbook*. Gower Medical Publishing, London.

Cook, R. I. and D. D. Woods 1994. Operating at the sharp end: the complexity of human error. In: *Human Error in Medicine* (M. S. Bognor, ed.), Lawrence Erlbaum Associates Publishers, Hillsdale, New Jersey.

Cooper, J. B., R. S. Newbower and R. J. Kitz (1984). An analysis of major errors and equipment failures in anaesthesia management considerations for prevention and detection. *Anaesthesiology*, **60**, 34-42.

Eagle, C. J., J. M. Davies and J. T. Reason (1992). Accident analysis of large scale technological disasters: applied to anaesthetic complications. *Canadian Journal of Anaesthesia*, **39**, 118-22.

Giraud, T., J. Dhainaut, J. Vaxelaire et al. (1993). Iatrogenic complications in adult intensive care units: a prospective two-centre study. *Critical Care Medicine*, **21**, 40-51.

HMSO. (1994). Report on confidential enquiries into maternal deaths in England and Wales. HMSO.

Hurst, N. W. and K. Ratcliffe (1994). Development and application of a structured audit technique for the assessment of safety management systems (STATAS). In Hazards XII European Advances in Process Safety. Institution of Chemical Engineers, Rugby.

Johnson, W. G. (1980). *Safety Assurance Systems*. Chicago: National Safety Council of America.

Leape, L. L. (1994). Error in medicine. *Journal of the American Medical Association*, **272**, (23), 1851-7.

Mills, D. H. (1995). Clinical risk management: experiences from the USA. In: *Clinical Risk Management* (C.A Vincent, ed.), British Medical Journal Publications, London.

Reason, J. T. (1993). The human factor in medical accidents. In: *Medical Accidents* (C. Vincent, ed.), Oxford Medical Publications, Oxford.

Reason, J. T. (1995). Understanding adverse events: human factors. In: *Clinical Risk Management* (C. Vincent, ed.), British Medical Journal Publishing Group, London.

Stanhope, N., C. A Vincent, S. E. Taylor-Adams, A. M. O'Connor and R. W. Beard (1997). Applying human factors methods to clinical risk management in obstetrics. *British Journal of Obstetrics and Gynaecology.* **104**, 1225-1232.

Swain, A. D. and H. E. Guttmann (1983). *A Handbook of Human Reliability Analysis with Emphasis on Nuclear Power Plant Applications.* NUREG/CR-1278. United States Nuclear Regulatory Commission, Washington DC, 20555.

Taylor-Adams, S. E., C. Vincent and N. Stanhope (1999). Applying Human Factors Methods to the Investigation and Analysis of Clinical Adverse Events. *Safety Science.* **31**, 143-159.

Vincent, C. and P. Bark (1995). Accident investigation: discovering why things go wrong. In: *Clinical Risk Management* (C. Vincent, ed.), British Medical Journal Publishing Group, London.

Vincent, C. 1997. Risk, Safety and the Dark Side of Quality. *British Medical Journal*, **314**, 1775-1776.

Vincent, C., S. E., Taylor-Adams and N. Stanhope (1998). Influences on clinical practice: a framework for the analysis of risk and safety in medicine. *British Medical Journal.* **316**, 1154-1157.

Williams, J.C. 1986. HEART - a proposed method for assessing and reducing human error. In 9th Advances in Reliability Technology Symposium, University of Bradford.

Wagenaar, J., J. Groeneweg, P. T. W. Hudson and J. T. Reason (1994). Safety in the oil industry. *Ergonomics*, **37**, (12), 1999-2013.

Wilson, R. M., W. B. Runciman, R. W. Gibber, B. T. Harrison, L. Newbyand and J. D. Hamilton (1995). The quantity in Australian health care study. *Medical Journal of Australia*, **163**, 458-71.

ACKNOWLEDGEMENTS

Dr Sally Adams would like to thank Healthcare Risk Resources International for funding her position at the Clinical Risk Unit. The authors would also like to thank Dr David Hewett (Medical Director, Winchester and Eastleigh Hospitals), Jane Chapman (Clinical Risk and Claims Manager, Northwick Park and St Marks Hospitals), Mr John Gray (Legal Services Manager, The United Bristol Healthcare NHS Trust), Sue Prior (Clinical Risk Manager, Winchester and Eastleigh Hospitals), Pam Strange (Patient Relations and Risk Manager, Bromley Hospital) and Anne Tizzard (Delivery Suite Manager, St Michael's Hospital) for assisting in the development of the framework and investigation process.

CHAPTER 7

ADVERSE EVENTS IN CARDIAC SURGERY: THE ROLE PLAYED BY HUMAN AND ORGANISATIONAL FACTORS

Jane Carthey*, Marc de Leval*, James Reason**, Andrew Leggatt* and David Wright***
*Cardiothoracic Unit, Great Ormond Street Hospital for Children, Great Ormond Street, London, WC1N 3JH.
**Psychology Department, The University of Manchester, Manchester, M13 9PL.
***Department of Statistical Science, University College London, London WC1E 6BT

INTRODUCTION

With ever increasing opportunities to carry out human factors research in medicine, there is a need to 'bridge the gap' between industry and the medical field. Existing human factors methods must be tailored for medical applications and human factors practitioners must appreciate the obstacles that they face when moving into this research domain. This chapter describes a human factors methodology for studying adverse events in paediatric cardiac surgery. A multi-centre study of neonatal arterial switch operations has been carried out, using a methodology based on Reason's (1990) organisational accident theory. This chapter discusses cultural problems associated with carrying out human factors research in medical domains, citing examples from paediatric cardiac surgery. Cardiac surgery is described as a high technology medical system which can be studied in the same way as other high technology domains. The methodology that was used in this study is described and some illustrative results are presented. The discussion focuses on our experience of carrying out human factors research in this area and the practical, methodological and data analysis problems that were experienced. It is concluded that human factors methods have an important role to play in understanding adverse outcomes in cardiac surgery.

'Bridging the Gap' Between Human Factors Research in Industry and Cardiac Surgery

Unlike the aviation and nuclear industries, there has not been a proliferation of human factors research in the field of cardiac surgery. Thus, there is a need to 'bridge the gap' that exists between cardiac surgery and other high technology industries. When one talks of 'bridging the gap between human factors research in industry and cardiac surgery' the most obvious question is what do we mean by 'a gap?' In the case of paediatric cardiac surgery, the human factors researcher is faced with cultural, knowledge, and language gaps that have to be bridged if research in this area is to be successful. These are described below:

The Cultural Gap. The cultural gap that exists between human factors research in industry and current medical thinking comprises four key elements:

- The notion of individual responsibility
- The blame culture
- Medico-legal pressures
- The attitudes and expectations of one's medical peers

From the perspective of individual responsibility, the clinician is viewed as, and himself feels, ultimately responsible for the wellbeing of his patient. For example, in cardiac surgery, when an adverse event occurs it is widely viewed as being due to an event that happened in the operating theatre, i.e. 'an operational hazard,' 'a surgical problem,' 'an anaesthetic problem.' Thus, adverse events in cardiac surgery have, prior to this study, been attributed solely to unsafe acts or active errors at the sharp end of the system, for example, in the operating theatre (Reason, 1990). There is a tendency to look only to the individual clinician for the causes of adverse events, which precludes attention being paid to the organisation itself.

The notion of individual responsibility, in conjunction with the medico-legal pressures that face the clinician when an adverse event occurs, leads to a 'blame culture', i.e. where there is a tendency to assign blame to whoever is deemed responsible for the adverse outcome. The blame culture permeates the belief that someone was '...at fault' for the adverse event to occur. Over time the blame culture decreases the potential to learn from error because people become wary of being blamed for an incident and therefore do not report adverse events.

The cultural gap between cardiac surgery and other high technology industries also manifests itself in people's attitudes, expectations and behaviour. The nuclear and aviation industries have to some extent accepted the inevitably of human error and strive towards making their systems error tolerant. In cardiac surgery the prevailing attitude and one that we have heard expressed many times during the course of our research is that 'a good surgeon should be able to cope with anything.' Thus, good surgeons should not fail. They are expected to cope with any scenario, irrespective of their level of surgical experience and whether or not they have encountered a similar situation in the past.

The legal pressures experienced in the medical field are another important component of the cultural gap that exists. Medico-legal cases reinforce the 'blame culture' that exists in medicine because they are driven by the aim of 'finding out who was at fault.' However, medico-legal cases trace back adverse events and are thus subject to hindsight bias. This means that all of the possible alternative courses of action that could have been taken at the time are easily seen with hindsight. Obviously, the clinician did not have this hindsight advantage at the time the adverse event occurred. He/she was more likely to be working under time pressure and trying to make accurate clinical decisions to ensure the best outcome for the patient.

The Knowledge Gap. The traditional approach to studying adverse outcomes in medicine is to look at the influence that patient and procedural variables had on the outcome of a case. For example, in the cardiac procedure that has been the focus of our research, the neonatal arterial switch procedure, it is well documented that an intramural course of the Left Anterior Descending coronary artery is associated with a higher risk of morbidity (Kirklin *et al.*, 1992). Research on the organisational and cultural antecedents of adverse events in cardiac surgery is sparse compared to other high technology industries.

In contrast to cardiac surgery, the nuclear power and aviation industries adopt a sociotechnical systems approach to accident analysis. Accident and incident analysis in these industries look beyond the active failures (Reason, 1990) that occurred at the task interface. They also investigate the organisational and cultural factors which created the preconditions for the accident to occur (See Figure 1). For example, analyses of the Chernobyl nuclear disaster have identified problems with the design of the RBMK reactor, and the management of the plant. These latent factors combined with the active errors made by the plant's operators to cause the accident (Reason, 1990).

However, tentative evidence pointing to the importance of the role of organisational and individual surgical performance on surgical outcomes does exist. From the perspective of organisational factors, it has been shown that there are differences between institutions in terms of the outcome of neonatal arterial switch cases (Kirklin *et al.*, 1992). In a multi-institutional study of risk factors associated with the neonatal arterial switch procedure, centres which had low mortality rates for this procedure at the start of the study were classified as 'low risk centres' (Norwood *et al.*, 1988). There were seven low risk centres in total. Eleven other centres were classified as 'high risk centres' on the basis of their high mortality rates at the start of the study (Norwood *et al.*, 1988). The institutional performance in the neonatal arterial switch operation was monitored over time. It was found that institutional performance in this procedure generally improved with increased institutional experience. However, two of the high risk centres had decreasing survival rates despite increased experience. Also, performance in one of the high risk centres improved more rapidly than in other high risk institutions. It was concluded that the observed differences with experience over time were due to, '... the differing institutional response to initially disappointing results.' (Kirklin *et al.*, 1992).

The role of the individual surgeon has also been highlighted. de Leval *et al.*, (1994) analysed the patient and procedural risk factors which influenced the outcome of a series of 104 neonatal arterial switch cases carried out by the same surgeon. After experiencing only one death in the first 52 patients in the series, 7 out of the next 16 patients died. The surgeon then elected to visit a low risk centre where the mortality rate for switch patients was low. The surgeon retrained in the switch procedure and, following the retraining, only one death occurred in the remainder of the series (i.e. only one death occurred in patients 69 to 104).

A logistic regression analysis of the patient and procedural risk factors was carried out to identify the key variables associated with risk. However, only half of the risk associated with the cluster of failures could be accounted for by the patient and procedural risk factor analysis. This led de Leval *et al.* (1994) to conclude that sub-optimal surgical performance at the time that the cluster of surgical failures occurred may have been the cause of the deaths. This factor seemed to have been neutralised by the surgical re-training process. de Leval *et al* (1994) also investigated whether monitoring 'near misses' (van der Schaaf, 1990) would have provided an earlier indication of a deterioration in surgical performance. This was the first application of the near miss concept to cardiac surgery. A near miss was defined as '...*the need to go back onto the heart lung bypass machine after the first attempt to wean the patient off bypass had failed (due to haemodynamic instability of the patient).*' Retrospective analysis of the data showed that if a near miss monitoring system had been in place prior to the cluster of failures, the surgeon would probably have been alerted that his performance was suboptimal.

To summarise, although there is tentative evidence that human and organisational factors account for differences in surgical outcomes, the nature of their influence and the underlying organisational and human processes that are important is not well understood in cardiac surgery. Thus, there is a significant knowledge gap that has to be bridged between human factors research and this surgical field.

The Language Gap. The cultural and knowledge gaps described above lead to language problems between the medical and the human factors field. Two factors are important here: Firstly, the paradigm difference in the way both fields look at adverse events makes it difficult for the human factors researcher and the cardiac surgeon to 'speak the same language.' Secondly, the human factors researcher's lack of medical knowledge is also important. If human factors research in any type of medical field is to be successful there is a need for the medical practitioners and human factors researchers to bridge the language gap. This involves a willingness on the part of the medical field to embrace human factors methodologies and an ability to acquire in-depth medical knowledge on the part of the human factors researcher.

Taken together, the cultural, knowledge and language gaps that exist between human factors research and cardiac surgery make it difficult to learn from adverse events. When adverse events occur, the cardiac surgeon wants to understand why and prevent a similar type of event occurring again. However, despite the motivation to learn from adverse events, the odds are stacked against the surgeon because of the cultural, knowledge and language barriers that exist. Taking cardiac surgery as an example of a broader problem in medicine, the cardiac surgeon exists in a 'blame culture', where the prevailing attitude is that good surgeons do not fail and the medico-legal implications of error are high. This cultural problem is further compounded by the knowledge and language problems that arise because human factors and medical analysis methods have thus far not been integrated. While the prevailing surgical culture means that learning about human factors may have a potentially high personal cost to the surgeon, the knowledge and language problems make it difficult to find appropriate methodologies. Together these problems create a strong tendency to maintain the status quo in cardiac surgery. A vicious circle ensues which leads to the focus of analyses on the patient and procedural factors that lead to adverse outcomes, to the neglect of the possible human and organisational causes.

CARDIAC SURGERY AS A HIGH TECHNOLOGY SYSTEM

The study described in the remainder of this chapter shows how the Catch 22 of medical culture can be overcome and how human factors and medical methodologies can be successfully integrated. A socio-technical systems approach to the analysis of adverse events in cardiac surgery has been developed, using Reason's theory of organisational accidents (Reason, 1990). Prior to outlining the methodology and some preliminary results of the study, cardiac surgery is described as a high technology system which can be studied from an organisational accident perspective.

Cardiac surgery is a high technology system which has common properties with the nuclear power and aviation industries. High technology systems are complex and tightly coupled (Perrow, 1983). They are characterised by dynamic problems where the situational conditions can change quickly and unexpectedly, sophisticated technology, complex human-machine interfaces and a complex social organisation of people who contribute specific types of expertise to ensure safe system performance. They also have high stakes of failure, where the margin for error is small and adverse events can lead to death or injury. A typical cardiac surgery organisation is described below to illustrate its classification as a high technology system.

The Structure and Characteristics of a Cardiac Surgery System

A cardiac surgery system comprises many different types of expertise. The decisions and actions carried out by the various system experts have to be co-ordinated to ensure the case has a good outcome. Furthermore, decision making authority is passed on from one subset of medical experts to another through the pre-operative, intra-operative and post-operative stages of patient care. The various types of expertise which have to be co-ordinated in a cardiac surgery system can be split broadly into three inter-dependent teams; the cardiology team, the theatre team and the intensivist team.

The Cardiology Team. The cardiology team is responsible for diagnosing the type of heart problem the patient has. They play an active role in the pre-operative planning of the case with the Consultant Surgeon and his team. The cardiology team also monitors the post-operative condition of the patient by carrying out regular echocardiogram tests on the heart while the patient is on the ward recovering from the surgical procedure. This team comprises one or more Consultant Cardiologist(s), senior registrars and senior house officer specialising in cardiology, echocardiogram staff, technicians and other support staff.

The Theatre Team. The theatre team is the principle team during the intra-operative stage of cardiac surgery, i.e. on the day the surgical procedure is carried out. The theatre team for paediatric open heart surgery comprises the following people; the Consultant Surgeon, Consultant Anaesthetist, Senior Surgical Registrar, Surgical Senior House Officer (SHO), Scrub Nurse and a perfusionist. There may also be a senior registrar in anaesthetics, who assists the Consultant Anaesthetist throughout the case.

The Intensive Care Team. The intensive care team comprises Consultant Intensivists, Consultant Cardiologists, Intensivist Registrars, nurses, physiotherapists, support technicians and others. This team is responsible for ensuring the stability and recovery of the patient following the surgical procedure.

Flexible Team Boundaries and Organisational Differences

An important point about cardiac surgery systems is that the team boundaries in the pre-operative, intra-operative and post-operative stages of the procedure are not completely fixed. Rather, they change according to the medical needs of the patient and can vary across different hospitals. For example, the cardiologist can become a member of the theatre team if the patient's condition requires that an intra-operative echocardiogram is carried out. Similarly, the Consultant Surgeon may be an important member of the cardiology team, depending on his expertise at reading ECHO's, the team relationships and the organisational structure of the hospital. Also, the role and level of decision making authority of the cardiology, surgical and intensivist teams varies across hospitals in the post-operative care of the patient. Whereas some intensive care units are led by the intensivist team, others are under the control of the Consultant Surgeon(s) or the cardiology team.

Sub-Teams Within Teams. Cardiac surgery systems are made more complex because they comprise 'sub-teams within teams'. This can be seen in the description of the theatre team roles given below. The theatre team has been chosen for a detailed description because the main focus of the research study reported later in this paper was the intra-operative care of the patient. The theatre team comprises the sub teams: surgical team, anaesthetic team and perfusion team.

The Surgical Team. The surgical team comprises the Consultant Surgeon, the senior surgical registrar, the senior house officer and the scrub nurse. The Consultant Surgeon has overall authority of the patient while in the operating theatre. He is the central decision maker in the theatre team, and is responsible for carrying out the surgical repair. The Consultant Surgeon also has several theatre team management tasks which require him to maintain a 'global overview' (Carthey, 1998) of the anaesthetic and perfusion aspects of the case. For example, the surgeon has to monitor the arterial blood pressure of the patient (on the ECG screen) to ensure that it does not drift up too high while the patient is on the heart lung bypass machine. The ECG is a piece of monitoring equipment that displays safety critical patient information. The other information which is usually displayed on the ECG screen is the electrocardiogram itself, the patient's heart rate, the left atrial pressure, the central venous pressure, the level of oxygen saturation in the blood, and the core and peripheral temperatures of the patient. These variables provide the Consultant Surgeon (and the rest of the theatre team) with abstract information on the condition of the patient's heart. The Consultant Surgeon integrates the abstract information from the ECG screen with visual information on the physical condition of the heart to form and update hypotheses about the patient's condition throughout the procedure.

The Senior Surgical Registrar. The Senior Surgical Registrar provides hands on assistance to the Consultant Surgeon throughout the case. The role of the senior registrar is to provide surgical support to the senior surgeon. This includes carrying out the sternotomy (i.e. opening the chest) at the start of the case, holding parts of the organ at the correct tension and in an appropriate position while the surgical procedure is being carried out and using the pump suckers to clear away blood in the heart cavity that may be obscuring the surgeon's view of the heart. The senior registrar is usually the most experienced of the two surgical assistants and is sometimes referred to as the 'first assistant.'

The Senior House Officer. The senior house officer is the second surgical assistant. Like the senior registrar, he is also responsible for holding parts of the organ at the correct level of tension and in the correct position throughout the procedure. He is also responsible for using the pump suckers to clear the blood from the chest cavity whenever this is appropriate.

The Scrub Nurse. The scrub nurse hands the surgical team the instruments that they need at appropriate points during the procedure. These instruments include cannulae (which are determined by the size and weight of the patient), suture lines, forceps, dissecting scissors, retractors and ice to cool the myocardium. Depending on her level of experience and the distribution of the surgical task workload, the scrub nurse may also have tasks which involve using the pump suckers to clear blood from the surgeon's view and holding parts of the organ at the correct tension and in the appropriate position.

An important part of the senior registrar's, surgical SHO's and scrub nurse's roles is the ability to anticipate the next part of the procedure before the surgeon actually does it. The anticipation of 'what the surgeon is going to do next' allows the two surgical assistants to position their hands and parts of the organ in an appropriate position. The scrub nurse's ability to anticipate future steps in the procedure gives her time to select the instruments that the surgeon will need and to be ready to hand them to him as required. The anticipatory behaviour of these three role types determines the degree to which the surgeon is able to maintain a constant 'surgical flow,' i.e. the uninterrupted progression of the surgical procedure. Thus, the tasks of the surgeon and the rest of the surgical team are tightly coupled, in the sense that the surgical flow of the procedure is dependent on each individual's ability to anticipate which procedural steps come next.

The Anaesthetic Team. The Consultant Anaesthetist intubates the patient and inserts venous and arterial lines at the start of the case. During the surgical procedure the Consultant Anaesthetist is responsible for tasks including administering the cardioplegia to the patient. (Cardioplegia is a potassium based solution which effectively freezes the heart and allows the surgeon to carry out the procedure on a stationary heart). The Consultant Anaesthetist's other tasks include setting up and administering the support drugs that are needed (usually inotropes like dopamine and dobutamine and vasodillators, e.g. glycerotrinitrate {GTN}), and monitoring the electrocardiogram screen. He/she may also be responsible for monitoring urine output and checking the coagulation levels of the blood (together with the perfusionist).

There is usually an anaesthetic registrar who assists the Consultant Anaesthetist during a case. Depending on the level of experience of the registrar, he will be delegated various anaesthetic tasks by the consultant anaesthetist. For example, the anaesthetic registrar may be asked to insert the neck line into the right jugular vein or to set up the support drugs in preparation for the patient being weaned from the heart lung bypass machine (see below).

Like the tasks within the surgical team, there is 'tight coupling' (Perrow, 1984) between anaesthetic and surgical tasks. For example, before the patient is put onto the heart lung bypass machine, the Consultant Anaesthetist must administer the anti-coagulant drug heparin. Heparin prevents the patient's blood coagulating in the heart lung bypass machine.

An omission error by the consultant anaesthetist at this stage in the procedure would result in an adverse event (i.e. a death or a near miss). Thus, the anaesthetic and surgical tasks are tightly coupled in the sense that the anaesthetist needs to know how far the surgeon has got with the pre-bypass surgical tasks to be able to decide when to administer the heparin. This information is gained by the anaesthetist observing the surgeon's pre-bypass surgical actions and through communication between the Consultant Surgeon and the consultant anaesthetist.

The Perfusion Team. During open heart surgery the heart is supported on a heart lung bypass machine. This piece of high technology hardware carries out the work of the heart and lungs during the surgical procedure. Prior to starting the surgical procedure, the patient is connected to the heart lung bypass machine via the insertion of arterial and venous cannulae into the heart. The heart lung bypass machine oxygenates venous blood and returns it to the patient via the arterial cannula. The perfusionist is the team member who controls this process. There are several important process variables which the perfusionist(s) has to monitor throughout the case, including the flow rate of the blood from the heart lung bypass machine to the heart, the coagulation levels of the blood, the oxygenation levels of the blood and the level of blood in the bypass machine reservoir.

The Consultant Surgeon depends on the perfusionist to regulate the level of blood flow between the heart lung bypass machine and the patient. The level of 'surgical visibility' (i.e. how good the surgeon's view of the heart is) throughout the case largely depends on how well the perfusionist does this task. There are also various points during the procedure when the coupling between the tasks of the perfusionist and the surgeon is critical to patient safety. For example, when the Consultant Surgeon is ready to go onto bypass he must communicate his readiness to proceed with this stage of the surgical procedure to the perfusionist. The perfusionist then has to start the flow of blood to the patient by removing the clamp from the arterial line of the heart lung bypass machine. This action allows the blood to flow to the patient's heart. Once the arterial blood flow to the patient has been established, the perfusionist and/or surgical assistants can remove the clamp on the venous cannula. This action starts the return flow of blood from the patient to the heart lung bypass machine. If the venous cannula clamp is removed prior to the arterial line clamp the patient will experience a heavy loss of blood, and in the worse case scenario may exsanguinate (i.e. bleed to death) on the operating table.

Similar types of inter-dependencies exist between the perfusion and anaesthetic tasks. For example, the perfusionist is able to administer certain drugs through the heart lung bypass machine (for example, isoflurane) and the anaesthetists need to know which drugs are being given in this way. This flow of information between the perfusionist and the anaesthetic team ensures that the perfusion and anaesthetic strategies are compatible.

STUDYING HIGH TECHNOLOGY CARDIAC SURGERY: AN ORGANISATIONAL ACCIDENT APPROACH

The preceding discussion has classified cardiac surgery as a high technology system which is complex and tightly coupled (Perrow, 1983). It follows from this classification that human factors theories that have been successfully applied to explain the genesis of accidents in other high technology systems (for example, the nuclear and aviation industries) could be used to understand adverse events in cardiac surgery. A multi-centre study looking at how human and organisational factors influence the outcomes of paediatric cardiac surgery was carried out, using Reason's (1990) organisational accident theory as a basis for the methodology. The neonatal arterial switch procedure was taken as a model of high technology cardiac surgery. This procedure is carried out on neonates who are born with transposition of the great arteries. The organisational accident theory that the methodology was based on is described below, followed by a layman's description of the neonatal arterial switch procedure. Following this the methodology of the study is outlined and some preliminary results are discussed.

Reason's (1990) Theory of Organisational Accidents

Reason (1990) has made a distinction between active and latent errors. Latent failures are those errors which result from fallible management decisions in the higher echelons of an organisation. Active failures are those unsafe acts which are committed by those at the immediate task interface. Latent failures lead to weaknesses in the organisation's defences and thus increase the likelihood that when active failures do occur they will combine with existing preconditions to breach the system's defences and result in an adverse event (see Figure 1). Thus, to properly understand the genesis of accidents one must understand both the latent and active errors that led to an accident.

This organisational theory of accident causation has been used to develop practical tools which pro-actively measure the 'safety health' of an organisation, i.e. to test how resilient it is to unsafe acts. These tools include TRIPOD, which has been developed for use in the off-shore oil industry and Managing Engineering Safety House (MESH), which has been used in the aviation industry.

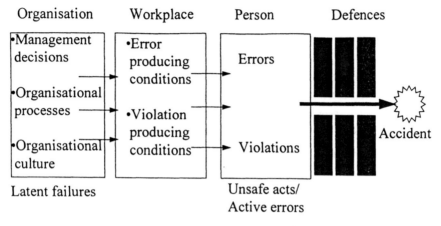

after Reason, 1990

Figure 7.1: Modelling organisational accidents

The Neonatal Arterial Switch Procedure: A Layman's Description

Patients who have transposed great arteries are born with an aorta that is connected to the right ventricle and the pulmonary artery connected to the left ventricle. Thus, the 'plumbing' of the heart is the opposite of that found in a normally developed heart. An 'arterial switch' procedure is carried out, usually in the first month of life. In the procedure the surgeon reconstructs the great vessels (i.e. the aorta and the pulmonary artery) so that the aorta is connected to the left ventricle and the pulmonary artery is connected to the right ventricle.

The patient is put on a heart lung bypass machine which does the work of the heart and lungs while the surgical procedure is carried out. The patient is cooled to approximately 18 degrees centigrade and the heart is 'frozen' using a potassium based substance called cardioplegia. The native aorta is transected. The coronary arteries are excised from the native aorta (i.e. the aorta which goes to the right ventricle) and re-implanted into the trunk of the native pulmonary artery (i.e. the vessel which is originally connected to the left ventricle). The coronary arteries are those blood vessels which carry blood from the aorta to the entire surface of the heart. These vessels are tiny in neonates (approximately 1 to 2 mm wide), so the surgeon has very little margin for error in the positioning of his sutures.

The re-implantation of the coronary arteries into the trunk of the native pulmonary artery creates a site which becomes the trunk of the new aorta, clinically termed the neo-aortic trunk. The neo-aortic trunk, with the newly re-implanted coronary arteries, is anastomosed (i.e. connected by means of suturing) to the descending aorta. Thus a new aorta is constructed which runs to the left ventricle.

In the next stage of the procedure, a piece of pericardium is used to reconstruct a neo-pulmonary artery trunk at the root of the native aorta (i.e. the original aorta that is connected to the right ventricle). The pericardium is the tissue that surrounds the heart. This is anastomosed to the ascending pulmonary artery and hence a new pulmonary artery is constructed that runs to the right ventricle. Clinically, this vessel is termed the neo-pulmonary artery. Following the reconstruction of the heart, the patient is re-warmed and weaned from the heart lung bypass machine. The patient is transferred to the intensive care unit after a period of haemostasis and when the electrocardiogram information shows that his condition is stable.

Human Factors and the Outcomes of Cardiac Surgery: The Neonatal Arterial Switch as a Model

All sixteen centres that carry out the neonatal arterial switch procedure in the United Kingdom (UK) have taken part in a study entitled, 'Human factors and the outcomes of cardiac surgery: The neonatal arterial switch as a model.' The switch procedure was chosen as a good model of high technology cardiac surgery because it reflects the high level of technical expertise which is needed on the part of the surgeon and the theatre team. The study involved the collection of three types of data:

Observations of Neonatal Arterial Switch Procedures. Data has been collected through on-site observations of neonatal arterial switch procedures. Prior to the start of the observational data collection, a detailed task analysis and a Failure Modes and Effects Analysis (FMEA) of the procedure was carried out. Failure Modes and Effects analysis involves breaking down a task into its component parts and using a set of 'error keywords' to identify the different types of problems that could occur in that task. During the analysis of the task, expert opinion is used to assess the likelihood that different types of errors will occur and the underlying causes of these errors. Finally, the consequences of the error for the overall safety of the system and the individual are described and, depending on the aims of the FMEA, a set of recommendations for improving the system are developed (see Kirwan and Ainsworth, 1992).

Task analysis and FMEA were tools used as part of a familiarisation process which allowed the human factors researchers to gain expertise of the procedure. Table 7.1 shows part of the Failure Modes and Effects analysis for the transfer of surgical information about the patient from the surgical team to the ICU team when the patient is handed over at the end of the case. At this point in the procedure several different types of communication failures can occur that all result in the ICU team receiving incomplete information on the patient's condition.

Table 7.1 shows only a subset of the problems that can be identified using this method (see Carthey *et al.*, 1999, for further examples).

Table 7.1

A Failure Modes and Effects Analysis Summary Table for Handover from the Theatre Team to ICU

Task	Failure Mode	Aetiology (active and latent causes)	Failure effect (i.e. consequences).
Communicate information on the surgical procedure to the ICU team.	Incorrect information communicated: Surgical assistant informs the ICU team that there has been an insignificant blood loss in the operating theatre when there has been a massive blood loss.	• Inaccurate understanding of the patients condition by the surgical assistant. • Inexperience of the surgical assistant. • Latent organisational policy problem; junior surgeon is left to hand over the patient alone.	ICU team are not primed to expect hypovolaemia and related problems.
Communicate information on the surgical procedure to the ICU team.	Information not communicated: No transfer of surgical information takes place.	• Time pressure on the surgical team to return to theatre to start the next case. • Last task in a long procedure effect. • Conflicting organisational demands; for example, the surgeon is needed in a meeting. • Misperception by the surgical team that ICU nurses do not need to know surgical details.	ICU team have incomplete information on the intra-operative events. ICU team are forced to seek the information they need which takes human resources away from patient care at a critical time.
Communicate information on the surgical procedure to the ICU team.	Communication too early: Surgical team communicate surgical information while ICU team are trying to set the patient up, set the electrocardiogram machine up and unravel the lines.	• Conflicting priorities of the ICU and surgical team. • Time pressure on the surgical team to return to theatre to start the next case. • Absence of a handover protocol.	ICU team do not receive critical patient information because it is delivered at a time when they are carrying out a higher priority task.

Observational data collection. A human factors researcher attended the neonatal arterial switch operations that were carried out over an 18 month data collection period (from January, 1996 to the end of June, 1997). The human factors researcher took written notes of what was happening from the start of the anaesthesia, throughout the entire surgical procedure and up until the patient had been handed over to the intensive care unit by the theatre team. These notes described the time an event happened and what actions were being carried out. During the surgical procedure the human factors researcher was either positioned on a platform looking over the surgeon's shoulder or at the front of the consultant anaesthetist's workstation. The human factors researcher recorded information on team relationships, surgical technique, goal handling, communication between the surgeon and his team, and any incidents or errors that occurred during the case. These included any minor events, for example, 'losses of surgical flow' that were caused by venous return problems or the surgical assistants not using the pump suckers to clear away blood that obscured the surgical visibility of the heart. Other types of minor event that were recorded included tension and positioning errors that were committed by the surgeons, 'external distracters', where people from outside the operating theatre team tried to communicate with the team during the case, delays in handing instruments to the surgeon by the scrub nurse, and communication problems between the surgeon and the rest of the theatre team. Information was also collected on a range of major events that occurred; these included major anaesthetic and surgical problems, for example, sub-optimal re-implantation of the coronaries. Following completion of the case the human factors researcher double checked his/her interpretation of any points that they were unsure of with the clinicians involved. The observer's notes were transcribed into a qualitative, written account of each case.

The observations were also used to collect information on the organisation itself. This information included the number of cases per annum, the number of surgical registrars and other staff, whether the centre was a dedicated paediatric cardiac hospital or a joint adult and paediatric centre, policy making in the organisation and any organisational problems thought to be important by the teams themselves.

Surgical Team Assessment Record (STAR). Secondly, self assessment questionnaires were filled in by members of the theatre team, using the Surgical Team Assessment Record (STAR). The STAR questionnaire allows each theatre team member to give their impression of how a range of organisational, team, situational, patient, procedural, personal and hand over (i.e. to ICU) factors influenced their performance during the case. STAR contains 34 items which each team member rates individually on a five point scale, ranging from -2 to +2. For example, each of the theatre team members described above would individually rate the personal factor 'mental readiness/preparedness' on this five point scale, depending on how they felt it affected them for case they had just carried out. The questionnaires were completed immediately after the patient had been transferred to the Intensive Care Unit. The respondents were the Consultant Surgeon, the Senior Surgical Registrar, Surgical Senior House Officer, the Scrub Nurse, the Consultant Anaesthetist and the perfusionist. Table 7.2 summarises all of the factors on the STAR questionnaire (see the following page).

Patient and Procedural Data. Finally, medical data on the patient and procedural variables was also collected. For example, the age, sex and weight of the patient, the types of drugs used during the anaesthesia, length of time spent on the heart-lung bypass machine, the length of time that the aorta is cross clamped, the coronary arterial pattern and specific aspects of the surgical procedure.

Data was collected on 230 neonatal arterial switch procedures in total. The data is being analysed using a logistic regression model which integrates the human, organisational, patient and procedural data and determines the relative contribution of each to adverse outcomes in cardiac surgery (de Leval *et al.*, 1999). The data analysis is still on-going and thus the full results of the study are currently unavailable. However, some preliminary insights from the observations are reported below.

Table 7.2

Factors Included in the STAR form

Category of Factors	Individual STAR Factors
Organisational Factors	Personnel availability Equipment availability Bed space in ICU Scheduling of the operation
Situational Factors	Free to concentrate/distractions and interruptions Physical conditions in the theatre 'Atmosphere' in the theatre Equipment design or reliability Monitoring of displays of equipment
Team factors	Pre-operative team briefings Confidence in other team members Team's ability to deal with unexpected events Communication between theatre teams Harmony/clashes between teams
Procedural Factors	Length of bypass Length of anaesthesia/lines insertion Length of the operation Accuracy of the diagnosis Drug administration
Patient Factors	Condition of the patient on arrival in anaesthesia Condition of the patient on arrival in theatre Condition after coming off bypass Condition on leaving the theatre
Personal Factors	Mental readiness/preparedness Keeping pace with events Technical performance Sleep/rest Well being/feeling off colour
Handover Factors (to ICU)	ICU readiness to receive the patient Communication between theatre team and ICU Equipment reliability during the handover Amount of time taken to handover Patients condition once fully monitored.

PRELIMINARY INSIGHTS FROM THE OBSERVATIONAL DATA ANALYSIS

Important insights into the genesis of adverse events in cardiac surgery have been gained from the case observations. Near misses and deaths in cardiac surgery can be modelled using the theory of organisational accidents (Reason, 1990), which has been described above, see Figure 7.1. Thus, adverse events in paediatric cardiac surgery can have a similar genesis to accidents in other high technology systems (i.e. the nuclear and aviation industries). Furthermore, the results have shown that some types of accident scenario recur. One particular type of 'generic accident scenario' has been identified which has repeatedly led to deaths and near misses. The term 'generic accident scenario' is deemed appropriate for these adverse events because, even though the specific circumstances of each case vary, they all have in common the same underlying general problems. The existence of generic accident scenarios in cardiac surgery suggests that, given certain latent preconditions, surgeons will experience similar types of problems at the surgical task interface.

The use of the 'near miss' concept (van der Schaaf, 1990) has also proven useful. The original definition of a near miss was, *'the need to go back onto bypass following the first period of weaning because of haemodynamic instability of the patient.'* (de Leval *et al.*, 1994). Several other types of near miss were identified, including cardiac arrest or cardiac tamponade[2] while the patient was in the intensive care unit. It was also noted that it was as important to study 'near miss avoidance' as near misses themselves. There were several cases when the actions of a member of the theatre team prevented a near miss from occurring. In one case the Consultant Surgeon was distracted two times by 'external distracters' during the pre-bypass surgical tasks. External distracters occur when the surgeon is asked to make decisions or provide information on clinical issues that are not related to the patient he is operating on. Non-theatre staff might come to the operating room and request information from the surgeon, thus interrupting the surgical flow of the procedure and distracting the surgeon from the task at hand. In this particular case, the surgeon was twice asked about the scheduling of the next day's cases by the operating theatre manager. These external distracters occurred just as the surgeon was preparing to put the patient onto bypass. The usual communication protocol for confirming that the heparin had been given was not initiated by the surgeon, who was expressing his annoyance at the interruptions. This communication protocol involves the surgeon asking the Consultant Anaesthetist (CA) to give the heparin and then waiting to receive confirmation that it has been given. The surgeon proceeded to insert the arterial cannula and informed the perfusionist that they would soon be ready to go onto bypass. At this point the Consultant Anaesthetist intervened and reminded the surgeon that the heparin had not been administered yet. Thus, the actions of the Consultant Anaesthetist may have prevented a near miss of going onto bypass prior to heparin administration. (However, it is important to note that the Consultant Surgeon had not yet inserted the venous cannula, so an important defence still had to be breached for this to happen).

Several different types of latent and active errors have also been identified. One of the most important 'latent errors' that occurs is an incorrect pre-operative diagnosis of the coronary arterial pattern. The coronary arterial pattern plays a large part in determining how complex the surgery will be, with highly abnormal patterns leading to increased surgical complexity. In addition to the latent errors that have been identified, several types of 'active error' have also been noted. For example, inexperienced surgeons tend to show 'cognitive lock up' (Sheridan, 1981) towards observing the physical symptoms from the heart and neglect to monitor the ECG screen. This can lead to adverse events where the condition of the patient deteriorates before the surgeon has realised that there is a problem.

DISCUSSION: THE LESSONS LEARNT FROM THIS STUDY

Being the first study of its kind to investigate the role played by human factors in cardiac surgery, many methodological issues were raised and lessons learnt during the research. The problems experienced were related to practical issues of carrying out human factors research in a medical domain, data collection and data analysis.

Practical Problems with Carrying out Human Factors Research in Medicine

Firstly, problems were experienced with ensuring the anonymity of the data because of its medico-legal implications. This was overcome by using a coding system to anonymise the responses on the STAR forms and the case study notes. Each member of the operating team, each centre and each case was given a numeric code to ensure that the data was anonymised.

The research team also faced the problem of how to ensure that their knowledge of the arterial switch procedure was sufficient to be able to make an informed assessment of each case. The transfer of expert knowledge to a novice is notoriously difficult at the best of times. In our case the problem was exacerbated by having novice researchers who, at the outset of the study, did not even understand the basics of medicine. Fortunately, the commitment and patience of the cardiac surgeon who had initiated the study won through; eventually a process of osmosis took place and a decent level of understanding was obtained by the research team. The learning curve was improved by the use of task and error analysis methods that allowed the human factors researcher(s) to break down the surgical procedure into its component parts and to understand it in their own terms. For example, the Failure

Modes and Effects analysis allowed failure modes associated with the component parts of the procedure to be broken down in a way the human factors team were familiar with.

Several data collection problems were also experienced. The original intention was to post off the STAR questionnaires to a designated person at each of the 16 hospitals involved in the study. This person would be responsible for handing out the forms and returning completed forms to the human factors team at Great Ormond Street Hospital. Pilot work showed that the only way to ensure a good response rate was for a human factors researcher to be present at each case. This had other benefits because the human factors researchers' observations of the cases proved to be a rich source of data that had not been envisaged in the initial research protocol. The data collection itself was a mammoth logistical task and its success was largely dependent on the good will of the surgeons involved in the study and their staff who were responsible for notifying the principal researcher every time a switch baby came into one of the units. The notification process was complex. There was a wide variety in the organisational structures of the centres and the person who was the most reliable source of information varied from centre to centre, from the Consultant Surgeon himself, the surgical secretary, the ICU nurses or other administrative and nursing staff who act as liaisons for external research projects. To ensure that the notification system worked effectively, we ensured that there was redundancy in the communication system, i.e. several contact people were asked to inform us when a switch baby came into the centre. The redundancy in our communications system meant that we were sometimes notified several times about one case, but we worked on the principle that as long as we were notified we were happy. The redundancy in the communication system also served us well during peak holiday times because it meant that we had enough cover to ensure that the notification system did not break down when key people were on holiday.

The data collection started on January 1st 1996; with the benefit of hindsight it would have been useful to have had a pilot month of data collection to test the communication system with the hospitals involved. In the post Christmas and New Year period people are not focused on starting new research projects and there were some teething problems with receiving notification from the hospitals at the start of the study.

Data Collection Problems

At the start of the study there was a feeling amongst some of the theatre team staff that the human factors researcher was '...the person carrying out the audit on switches.' The initial anxieties that people had about taking part in the study were overcome in a variety of ways. Each centre was visited by the principal researcher prior to the start of the data collection. This informal visit allowed the researcher to meet as many people as possible and introduce the research to them on a one-to-one basis. This gave hospital staff the opportunity to express any concerns that they had and to iron these out prior to the data collection starting in earnest. During this visit, and through subsequent visits, the aim of the study was described as a shared learning opportunity for everyone, not a test of an individual's performance.

There was a limited window of opportunity to collect the STAR data. The STAR questionnaires had to be completed as soon after the case as possible and the human factors researcher had to keep track of where each individual in the theatre team went to after leaving the operating theatre. We soon realised that there are a myriad of places to hide in a hospital! The theatre team were often needed back in the operating theatre to carry out a second (or third) case, the surgeons and anaesthetists sometimes had meetings to attend or other patients to see between cases, so it was important to judge the appropriate time to hand out the STAR form and to ask for the completed form back.

For the case study observations we chose to record what was going on rather than to have a pro forma where the team were rated on a series of key factors (for example, Helmreich *et al.* 1995). This meant that it was important for the human factors researcher to position herself so that she had a good view of the surgical procedure throughout, but at the same time be an unobtrusive observer.

Data Analysis Problems

Important lessons have also been learnt from the data analysis. The statisticians faced the problem of integrating the 'hard data', i.e. the clinical data with the subjective impressions of the theatre team on the STAR form. This was achieved by developing a baseline logistic regression model using clinical factors and adding the STAR data to this model. In the third phase of the analysis, data from the case studies were added to the regression model (see de Leval *et al.*, 1999, for a full discussion). The main problem that occurred during this stage of the analysis was the large number of variables that could have potentially been included in the data analysis as opposed to the number of cases that were observed (i.e. n=230). To carry out a meaningful statistical analysis the data was collapsed in a variety of ways, for example, STAR factors were collapsed into organisational, situational, team, personal, patient and procedural categories. There were too few responses for the 'handover factors' part of the questionnaire to carry out a statistical analysis on this section of the STAR form. This finding reflects the wide variation in handover practices across the different centres, where there are differences in the theatre staff who have responsibility for handing the patient over to the intensive care unit team. Finally, the overall responses on the STAR form indicated that theatre staff live in a 'toleration culture' where they accept a range of human and organisational problems as a way of life. The theatre teams perceived many of the factors on the STAR form as everyday events that they had no control over and which they were willing to tolerate as long as the case had a good outcome. An important limitation with the STAR data is the effect that the knowledge of the outcome of the case influenced the ratings on the STAR form, given that this 'toleration culture' exists.

A further data analysis problem was that some of the centres and surgeons taking part in the study are 'low volume' centres/surgeons who carry out less than 10 switch procedures per year. This meant that the data had to be pooled into 'low volume', 'medium volume' and 'high volume' centres/surgeons and that individual analysis of each centre's and surgeon's results was not possible. However, this problem was anticipated at the outset of the study and the aim was not to test the results of individual surgeons.

Like all research that uses case study data, we also faced the problem of how best to analyse it so that it was consistent, reliable and so that valid conclusions could be drawn. The human factors researchers' knowledge of the switch procedure was an iterative process and to ensure consistency and reliability in the qualitative data analysis some of the earlier case study notes were eliminated in the analysis stage. This meant that only those cases where the researcher was judged to have attained a good understanding of the surgical procedure were used. Generally, the case study data that had been collected by the two principal HF researchers was good quality, and a wide range of human factors problems were identified. Two levels of analysis are being carried out on the case study data:

1. An error analysis, where all of the problems and errors that were experienced in each case are categorised. This analysis will allow comparisons between surgeons /centres for the frequency of different types of errors and problems that occur during their cases.

2. An 'excellence' analysis, where a framework of the factors that underpin surgical excellence has been developed and used to rate each of the cases. This framework has been described in detail in Carthey, *et al.* (1999).

CONCLUSION

Medical research typically focuses on how patient and procedural factors lead to adverse outcomes. There is a need to integrate human factors methodologies into medical research to examine the human and organisational factors that contribute to adverse events. This chapter has described a study that has integrated human factors into a high technology medical domain: paediatric cardiac surgery. Various methodological problems have been discussed and hopefully some of the lessons that have been learnt in this study will prove useful to other research teams. The study itself marks the advent of a cultural shift in the way that UK paediatric cardiac surgeons investigate the causes of adverse events. However, it is only a small step in the right direction towards bridging the gap that currently exists between medical domains and other high technology industries in terms of how they understand negative events. Future research is needed that develops more refined human factors methodologies to investigate other medical domains and which enhances the preliminary insights into paediatric cardiac surgery that have resulted from this study.

REFERENCES

Carthey, J. (1998). *Communication and decision making in nuclear emergencies: A field study.* Unpublished PhD manuscript. Client confidential. Industrial Ergonomics Group, The University of Birmingham, UK.

Carthey, J., M. R de Leval, J. T. Reason, D. Wright and A. Leggatt (1999). Human factors and cardiac surgery: Identifying the problems and positive aspects of surgical performance. In press: To be published in the *Proceedings of the International Conference on Improving Patient Safety and Reducing Errors in Healthcare,* November 8-10, 1998. Rancho Mirage, California, USA. The National Patient Safety Foundation, Chicago. Ill. USA.

de Leval, M., K. Francois, C. Bull, W. Brawn and D. Speigelhalter (1994). Analysis of a cluster of surgical failures: Application to a series of neonatal arterial switch operations. *The Journal of Thoracic and Cardiovascular Surgery,* March.

de Leval, M. R., J. Carthey, D. J.Wright, V. T. Farewell and J. T. Reason (1999). Human factors and surgical outcomes: A multi-centre study. Paper presented at the 79th Annual Meeting of The American Association of Thoracic Surgery, April 18-21st, 1999, New Orleans, USA. In press, to be published in *The Journal of Thoracic and Cardiovascular Surgery,* 1999.

Helmreich, R. L., H. G. Schaefer and J. B. Sexton (1995). Operating Room Checklist (ORC), NASA/UT/FAA Technical Report 95-4, Austin, TX: The University of Texas.

Kirklin, J W., E. Blackstone, C. Tchervenkov, A. Castenada and the Congenital Heart Surgeons Society (1992). Clinical outcomes after the arterial switch operation for transposition: patient, support, procedural and institutional risk factors. *Circulation,* **86,** 1501-1515.

Kirwan, B. and L. Ainsworth (1992). *Task analysis: A users guide.* Taylor and Francis.

Norwood, W. I., A. R. Dobell, M. D. Freed, J. W. Kirklin, E. H. Blackstone and The Congenital Heart Surgeons Society (1988). Intermediate results of the arterial switch operation. *Journal of Thoracic and Cardiovascular Surgery,* **96,** 854-862.

Perrow, C. (1983). *Normal accidents: Living with high risk technologies.* Basic Books, New York.

Reason, J. (1990). *Human Error*. Cambridge University Press.

Van der Schaaf, T. W., D. A. Lucas and A. R. Hale (1991). *Near miss reporting as a safety tool*. Butterworth Heinemann Ltd. Oxford.

Sheridan, T.B. (1981). Understanding Human Error and Aiding Human Diagnostic Behaviour in Nuclear Power Plants. In: *Human Detection and Diagnosis of System Failures* (J. Rasmussen and W.B. Rouse, eds.), pp.119-135. Plenum Press, New York.

ACKNOWLEDGEMENTS

The research team would like to thank the 21 cardiac surgeons and their staff for their co-operation and enthusiasm during this study. This research was supported by The British Heart Foundation, whose support we would also like to acknowledge. Special thanks go to Roisin Baldwin, Jenny Porter and Jackie Banfield, the three medical secretaries in the Cardiac Unit at Great Ormond Street Hospital, for their contribution and support.

CHAPTER 8

ENHANCING TEAM PERFORMANCE

Stephan C.U. Marsch, Christoph Harms, Daniel H. Scheidegger, Department of Anaesthesia, University of Basel, Switzerland

INTRODUCTION

Operating rooms, intensive care units, or emergency rooms are domains designed for the care of the acutely ill high-risk patient. The medical problems encountered by health care professionals working in these domains are highly complex. This is due to the inherent complexity of many problems, and the limited time available, thus making successful management clearly beyond the capacity of a single practitioner. Consequently, a team approach rather than a single practitioner based approach is required in high-risk medical domains.

Common sense would suggest that the quality of team performance has an impact on patients' outcome. However, this topic has seldom been formally addressed by research, and we know little about how the performance of medical teams can be enhanced. There is, however, anecdotal evidence of the importance of team performance: every healthcare professional involved in high-risk medical endeavours has experienced examples of poor team performance leading to disasters and good team performance leading to good outcome in critical situations.

EXAMPLES OF TEAM PERFORMANCE

The most impressive examples of poor team performance in the operating room are operations performed on the wrong side of the body (mixing up of left and right side), or on the wrong patient (mixing up of patients). One could argue that the surgeon performing the operation is ultimately responsible for such a disaster. This view, however, is too simplistic. In one such case, an anaesthesiologist, who had visited the patient prior to the operation, was present from the moment the conscious patient entered the operating room until the start of the operation; an orderly positioned the patient for his operation on the operating table; a scrub nurse disinfected the skin overlying the site of the intended operation and covered the patient with sterile drapes. Thus, any of the health care professionals present in the operating room could have prevented the surgeon from performing the wrong operation. We would consider therefore that the occurrence of such an error to be a failure of a complete operating room team, rather than a failure of a single person who is unfortunate enough to perform the last and decisive step in a complex chain of events.

Doctors Fined for Fight in Operating Room

Worcester, Mass. Nov. 27 (AP)

--- A state medical board has fined a surgeon and an anesthesiologist $ 10,000 each for brawling in an operating room while their patient slept under general anesthesia. After their fight, the anesthesiologist Dr. Kwok Wie Chan, and the surgeon Dr. Mohan Korgaonkar, successfully operated on the elderly female patient. In addition to imposing the fines, the state board of Registration in Medicine last week ordered the doctors to undergo joint psychotherapy. It also directed officials at the Medical Center of Central

Massachusetts, who had already put the doctors on five years' probation, monitor Drs. Chan and Korgaonkar for five years. The medical board said that on Oct. 24, 1991, Dr. Korgaonkar was about to begin surgery when he and Dr. Chan began to argue. Hospital officials would not provide the nature of their disagreement. Dr. Chan swore at Dr. Korgaonkar, who threw a cotton-tipped prep stick at Dr. Chan, the board said. The two then raised their fists and scuffled briefly, at one point wrestling on the floor. A nurse monitored the anesthetized patient as the doctors fought.

Figure 8.1. Conflict in the operating room.

Conflicts are another source of poor team performance, though few are as overt as that depicted in figure 8.1. More subtle and/or unresolved conflicts may result in individuals being distracted from their task. Moreover, unresolved conflicts may result in team members not expressing their concerns when they should. For example, during hip arthroplasty for a fractured femoral neck, a surgeon in a Swiss hospital misplaced the saw and cut away too much of the femoral bone. This resulted in major difficulties in completing the operation and exposed the patient to a significant additional perioperative risk because of prolonged intraoperative bleeding. In addition, the ultimate goal of the operation, enabling the patient to walk, was seriously threatened. The scrub nurse later admitted that she was fully aware of the misplacement of the saw and that she could have easily prevented the error. However, having been "tormented" by this surgeon for years she felt that his error "would serve him right" and did not intervene.

The importance of good team performance becomes fully apparent in critical situations in which rapid and effective action is required by all members of the team. These critical situations may arise due to the patient's condition, technical malfunction, or even human error. After a car accident, an otherwise healthy patient was scheduled to have internal stabilisation of his fractured cervical spine in the prone position. During the operation an accidental extubation occurred, i.e. the plastic tube connecting the patient's trachea with the respirator slipped out of the trachea. This resulted in a potentially fatal incident because the patient could no longer be oxygenated and nothing could be done to improve the situation in the prone position. The operating room team was faced with the complex task of turning a patient with an open wound in the neck and an unstable cervical spine from the prone into the supine position. This task had to be accomplished as quickly as possible to ensure oxygenation and hence the survival of the patient. However, the unstable cervical spine required a careful approach to avoid damage to the cord, with the prospect of complete tetraplegia as the worst possible outcome. An outstanding team performance, based on excellent communication, task prioritisation, and clear workload distribution ensured a favourable outcome: the patient was turned in the supine position, re-intubated, and, after the airway had been secured, turned back into the prone position to enable the completion of his operation. The remainder of the operation was uneventful and the patient left the hospital without any signs or symptoms of hypoxic brain damage or damage to the cervical cord.

Risk to Patients

Any discussion of team performance and quality of care needs to be set in the broadest context of the overall scale of errors and adverse events in healthcare. Modern healthcare has become a very complex endeavour that involves interactions between patients and many different health care professionals. Each interaction presents an opportunity for mistakes and errors which in turn may result in accidental injury. Each accidental injury may result in significant morbidity and even mortality.

The medical, social, and economic impact of accidental injuries in hospitalised patients is enormous: the Harvard Medical Practice Study reported that nearly 4% of patients hospitalised in the state of New York in 1984 suffered an unintended iatrogenic injury, defined as prolongation of hospital stay or measurable disability at the time of discharge (Brennan *et al.*, 1991). Sadly, more than 70% of these adverse events were, retrospectively, classified as preventable (Leape *et al.*, 1991).

Despite the mounting evidence of the epidemic proportion of medical-care induced adverse events in the 1980s (Perper *et al.*, 1994), most medical specialties have not formally addressed this issue. One significant exception is anaesthesia, which has evolved as the leading medical speciality when it comes to issues like patient safety, critical incidents, or risk management: Cooper *et al.* (1978) identified human error as the leading cause of anaesthesia-related complications. Their findings were confirmed by the largest survey on anaesthesia-related incidents conducted so far: Williamson *et al.* (1993) demonstrated that human error was either the main cause or significantly contributed to more than 70% of 2000 critical incidents. Moreover, more than 60% of the incidents were classified, retrospectively, as preventable. As far as intensive care is concerned, Donchin *et al.* (1995) estimated that a severe or potentially detrimental error occurs on average twice per patient per day. In addition, Cullen *et al.* (1997) reported an incidence of 19 preventable adverse drug events per 1000 patient days in intensive care. The role of team performance in such events, however, has yet to be elucidated.

TEAM WORK IN HIGH-RISK MEDICAL DOMAINS

Heterogeneity in Medical Teams

Compared to other high-risk domains, teams in the operating room, the intensive care unit, and the emergency room are particularly complex and heterogeneous groups. Team members differ in their profession (e.g. surgeon, anaesthetist, scrub nurse), but also in professional education (academic, non-academic), hierarchy (consultant, resident) and status. Gender too is an issue as, at least in our country, most nurses are female while the majority of doctors are male. Moreover, healthcare workers are organised in different subdivisions of the hospital (e.g. department of anaesthesia, department of surgery, department of nursing). Each of these subdivisions has its own distinct culture of shared values, norms, and rituals. Members of teams in high-risk medical domains therefore differ not only in personality, but also in profession, professional education, and cultural background.

As far as operating teams are concerned, there is a basic division into two major subgroups: the anaesthetic team and the surgical team. All issues relevant for team performance in a high-risk environment (e.g. communication, leadership) play an important role not only within both subgroups but also at the interface between both teams. Most of the tasks required to perform a safe operation are clearly divided between the two teams. There is, however, an overlap in some tasks and the degree of responsibility for shared duties may vary between the teams depending on the type and time course of surgery.

Working Conditions

Working conditions for healthcare workers in the operating room, intensive care, and emergency medicine resemble those of high-risk environments such as aviation rather than those of other medical specialities. As in other high-risk technological domains (aviation, nuclear power station) operating rooms, intensive care units, or emergency rooms are highly complex environments. Typical features of working conditions include uncertainty, rapid changes in the patient's condition, and intense time pressure. In addition, the ergonomic working conditions are often less than ideal. The technological reliability and sophistication is such that the occurrence of disasters due to failure of equipment is extremely rare. Instead, the patient's condition and human errors are the main cause of critical incidents and adverse outcomes.

ENHANCING TEAM PERFORMANCE IN HIGH-RISK MEDICAL DOMAINS

Scope of Measures Intended to Enhance Team Performance

Human error is the most important cause of critical incidents in the operating room, in intensive care, and in the emergency room. However, the skills of healthcare workers are the last defence against the consequences of technical failure, equipment malfunction and unexpected complications and, in most of the cases, only human beings are capable of mitigating the consequences of human error. Thus, human performance in high-risk medical environments is at one and the same time the weakest, and hence most dangerous, link in the treatment chain as well as the last and most powerful resource for preventing accidents. Any policy to enhance team performance should focus on both aspects of the human role in the high-risk medical domain: healthcare workers must realise that they are the major source of potentially preventable adverse events. On the other hand, healthcare workers must also realise that their performance in critical situations can be the deciding factor in preventing an unfavourable outcome.

How to Assess Team Performance?

Many practitioners know the rewarding feeling of being part of a good team with a high level of performance. Some also know the rather unpleasant experience of realising that one is part of a team that performs poorly. Observers of teams, be it in the medical field or in other domains (e.g. sport), usually have no difficulty in rating a team's performance as outstanding, good, or poor. However, it is quite difficult to define the key elements of team performance that lead to such ratings and to the impression of being part of a good or poor team. The rating of team performance in medicine is often based on subjective criteria or 'gut feeling' rather than scientifically sound parameters.

To assess team performance in aviation, researchers of the University of Texas have developed the LINE/LOS checklist (Helmreich and Merritt 1998). LINE stands for observations during normal flight operations while LOS stands for Line Operational Simulation, i.e. full mission simulation. This checklist defines observable actions that have been implicated in accidents or incidents. However, these standards were developed for the U.S. aviation community and cannot simply be copied for the use in a different culture or a different professional domain. As outlined above, the situation in the operating room is much more complex than that in the cockpit. Thus, it is not clear whether team performance markers designed to assess the performance of a team of two pilots are suitable to assess within and between team communication in the operating room.

Our group has adapted and modified the LINE/LOS check-list in order to assess team performance in the operating room. As a first step, we were able to demonstrate feasibility and reproducibility of observing operating room teams in routine clinical practice (Sexton *et al.*, 1998a). However, as yet no proper validation of the checklist has been performed and the effects of cultural and organisational factors remain to be determined. Thus we have to realise that in most areas of medicine there is presently no validated tool available to assess team performance. This is a major problem since it is impossible to reliably determine the impact of measures taken to improve team performance.

Improving Team Performance by Team Training?

How can we train teams to commit fewer errors? Experience from aviation suggests that team formation, leadership, communication and workload distribution are critical for a safe team performance. We believe that these issues are equally important in high-risk medical domains. Our hypothesis is that teams capable of building and maintaining a good group climate that encourages participation and exchange of information will commit fewer errors, will retrieve more errors, and will be more successful in mitigating the consequences of errors and unforeseeable complications.

How can we train teams to be more effective in the management of unexpected critical situations? Again, there is little data on this topic in the medical field or in other high-risk domains. For example, it is not known whether team performance at a normal workload predicts team performance in a subsequent critical incident. It is not inconceivable that teams performing poorly at times "when it doesn't matter" may rise to the occasion if they need to. We believe however, that a pre-existing good team climate facilitates the management of critical incidents. Maintenance of a high level of team performance at all times should thus be the final goal of any institutional policy aiming to enhance team performance.

Outcome Measures

While most healthcare professionals would probably agree that the quality of team performance is important for patients' safety, overall quality of care and staff morale, there is little scientific evidence to support this view. A crucial initial question for researchers is the designation of appropriate process or outcome measures against which team performance can be judged. A reduction in preventable mortality would be the strongest indication for the success of measures implemented to improve team performance. However, the perioperative mortality is presently quite low (approximately 1:10'000). We estimated that, for reasons of sufficient statistical power, more than half a million patients had to be included in a study designed to show that enhancing team performance results in a 50% decrease in mortality. This number is beyond the scope of any single institution and would require a multi-centre approach. Aviation is facing a similar problem. Most pilots and airlines agree that Crew Resource Management (CRM), a simulator based training aiming to improve team performance in the cockpit, enhances flight safety. However, due to the low incidence of crashes of civil aircrafts the success, if any, of CRM in reducing accidents cannot be directly demonstrated.

The number of critical incidents could serve to indicate the success of programmes aiming to enhance team performance. However, neither the definition nor the detection of critical incidents is straightforward. Moreover, the implementation of team training within an organisation may, directly or indirectly, change the organisational culture as far as safety is concerned. This might lead to a larger number of incidents being disclosed that otherwise would not have been noticed or even been hidden from management. Thus, successful team training may even lead to an apparent increase in critical incidents.

In times of mounting economic pressure on the healthcare system, the question arises as to whether the quality of team performance has an impact on issues like efficiency. Common sense would indicate that better teams make better use of their resources. There is presently no data available supporting this view, but measures of efficiency, such as the time taken to complete standards tasks, could certainly be used as one indicator of team performance.

The Importance of the Institution

What is required to ensure a high level of team performance within an institution? The medical field relies heavily on a strong hierarchy. Thus, any policy aiming at enhancing team performance needs the endorsement of the top hierarchical level. In fact, only if the chairmen and senior staff of all departments involved accept and actively support the measures taken can such a programme succeed. Verbal commitment alone is clearly insufficient. In order to become successful, any programme designed to enhance team performance needs institutional support. In addition, most, if not all, institutions aiming to improve team work within their boundaries need to undergo a change in culture. For example, the mere fact of addressing behavioural issues may be perceived as a threat to one's own personality and privileges and so inspire fear and rejection at any level of the organisation.

The existing training of healthcare workers concentrates on the technical skills of individuals. Thus, as a first step, individuals training to enhance team performance have to be made aware of the importance of team work and some of the key markers of good team performance. Lectures and seminars may be suitable tools to achieve this purpose. As a second step, individuals have to learn to work as members of a team. Such training can be conducted 'on the job' by senior staff or in the simulator. In the aviation community Crew Resource Management, a simulator-based training, has become an invaluable tool to improve skills in human factors and team issues (Helmreich and Foushee, 1993).

THE UNIVERSITY OF BASEL APPROACH

Increasing awareness of the importance of human factors and team performance in the Department of Anaesthetics at the University of Basel in Switzerland has led to a variety of activities. Most notably, an operating room simulator has been built. A cornerstone of our efforts is the co-operation of the Departments of Anaesthetics, Nursing, and Surgery that enables all healthcare workers normally involved in the care of the patient in the operating room to take part in the simulator training.

Team Orientated Medical Simulation (TOMS)

Team orientated medical simulation (TOMS) involve a high-fidelity full scale simulation of a complete operating room, including all personnel usually involved in patient care (Marsch et al., 1999). This novel approach to training in the medical field was invented by a research team led by the late Hans-Gerhard Schäfer MD and first performed at the University of Basel in Switzerland in December 1994. The main purpose of TOMS was to adapt and implement the concepts of CRM for complete operating room teams.

The simulator is situated on the hospital campus remote from the building housing the operating theatres. The simulator is essentially a room that has been transformed into an operating theatre and which allows high-fidelity simulation of surgery and anaesthesia (figure 8.2). In order to make the simulations as realistic as possible all equipment used in the simulator is, whenever possible, identical to that used in the real operating room. The anaesthetic part of the patient consists of a resuscitation mannequin. The mannequin can be intubated and mechanically ventilated. Both venous and arterial access can be established and used for administering fluids and drugs or monitoring of the patient respectively. ECG, invasive and non-invasive blood pressure, and oxygen saturation are controlled by software and displayed on a commercially available anesthesia monitor.

In the majority of simulations we use a laparoscopic simulator for the surgical task, which essentially consists of a plastic box covered by a rubber top to allow the penetration of laparoscopic instruments. Laparoscopic surgery is performed on porcine organs obtained from the slaughterhouse. Most simulations conducted so far required the surgeons to perform a laparoscopic cholcystectomy. Alternative scenarios include abdominal aortic repair, performed on a specially designed plastic model, and surgical repair of bone fractures.

All personnel usually involved in the care of the patient in the real operating theatre take part in a simulation. This includes the anesthetic team (anesthetic nurse, resident anesthetist, staff anesthetist) and a surgical team (scrub nurse, orderly, resident surgeon, staff surgeon). On the day of simulation one regular operating room remains closed so that personnel can be shifted to the simulated operation. It was agreed that our organisation could afford one simulation day every month, each involving two simulator sessions (morning and afternoon).

The simulation session consists of three parts: briefing, simulated operation, and debriefing. During the briefing, participants are informed of the aims of the training session. Confidentiality and the intention to train and learn, rather than to evaluate, are especially emphasised. This is followed by a technical briefing that focuses on the equipment available and the technicalities of the simulator. The task of the team during the following simulation is to perform surgery as scheduled on a mannequin under general anesthesia. Our scenarios are not designed to test the technical skills of the individual participants. In addition, we deliberately aim at a normal or moderately increased work load. Our intention is not to force the team to work beyond the limits of their capabilities. Instead, we intend to simulate a 'routine operation'. This allows the participants to concentrate on issues related to human factors and experiment with 'new' behaviour. Simulation sessions are videotaped. Besides the visual information, the videotapes contain recordings of wireless microphones attached to every participant.

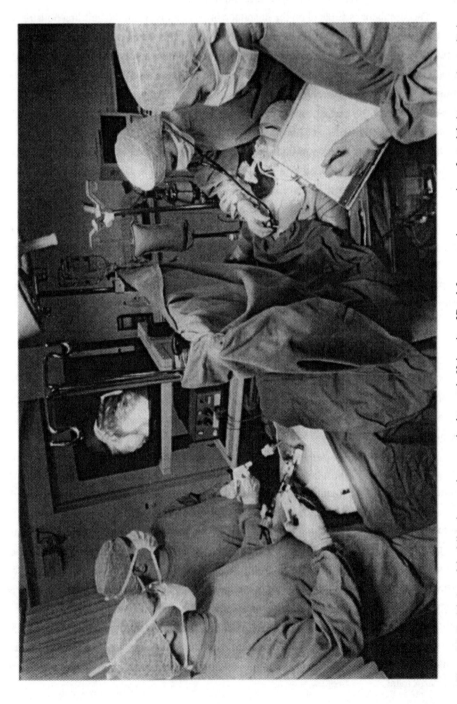

Figure 8.2. Partial view of the full scale operating room simulator at the University of Basel. Laparoscopic surgery is performed during general anaesthesia.

During the debriefing, videotapes are reviewed by all participants. Sequences are selected by the instructor to highlight typical behavioural patterns and, in addition, participants may request specific events to be displayed and discussed. The debriefing should be an interactive event and participants are encouraged to share their experiences during simulation. An important part of the debriefing session is discussion of the implications, if any, of team performance experienced during simulation for the 'real' operating room.

Achievements of TOMS

One of the major achievements of TOMS was its actual implementation. Within our institution three independent departments (surgery, anaesthesia, nursing) had to agree that joint simulations should be carried out. Moreover, it was agreed to close one operating theatre one day a month and perform simulations with the staff scheduled for that theatre. Despite many problems regular simulations were carried out without interruption over a period of four years.

Simulations with complete operating room teams achieved a high level of perceived realism of team behaviour. Figure 8.3 shows participants' rating of the realism of team behaviour as compared with the real operating room on a 10 point Lickert scale (1 = completely unrealistic, 10 = completely realistic). The median scale was 8 with no statistically significant difference among the different subgroups (Sexton *et al.*, 1998b). These favourable ratings occurred despite problems with surgical scenario that are outlined in the following paragraph.

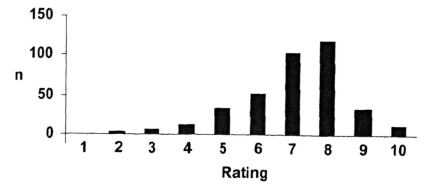

Figure 8.3. Participant's rating of the perceived realism of team behaviour during simulator training of complete operating room teams. A 10 point Lickert scale is used: 1 = completely unrealistic as compared to the real operating room, 10 = completely realistic as compared to the real operating room.

Observations performed in the real operating room prior to the start of TOMS demonstrated that team behaviour, and especially communication, was less than ideal (Sexton *et al.*, 1998a): in about 20% of operations team performance was rated to be below standard. Observations are currently being made to assess whether and how the simulation training affected team performance in the real operating room. Preliminary results suggest a trend towards improved ratings for areas like communication and conflict management (Marsch *et al.*, 1999).

Problems encountered with TOMS

In all new endeavours problems are inevitable and TOMS is no exception. Two major problems became apparent during the last two years. First, shortage of personnel in all departments involved made the planning of the simulations increasingly difficult. Moreover, shifting human resources from the real operating room to the simulator led to conflicts, especially in times of high workload. Second, the surgical scenarios available proved to be not interesting enough for the surgeons involved. Indeed, both our scenarios (laparoscopic cholecystectomie and abdominal aneurysm repair) offered only a limited range for simulated complications. Consequently, our surgeons rated the scenarios as not challenging enough, reducing their perceived benefit of participating in simulator sessions. This resulted in surgeons 'excusing' themselves from scheduled sessions and senior surgeons forcing their junior colleagues to replace them in the simulator. We became convinced that conflicts provoked by continuing our programme would more than annihilate its benefits, if any, and we decided provisionally to stop regular simulations at the end of 1998. Whether we will be ever able to resume training complete operating room teams in the simulator is presently uncertain.

Another important lesson learned was that the primary interest of most, if not all, participants did not relate to team issues. Instead, participants expect to gain an individual benefit from the simulation, such as enhancing their skills or testing their abilities. This by no means indicates that participants did not appreciate good team work. In contrast, most participants rated the importance of communication as high and agreed that behavioural issues were a key determinant of team performance in the operating room. However, the primary motivation to participate in the simulation appeared to be individual benefit. Under these circumstances, the key to a successful simulation programme is the design of scenarios that are challenging on an individual level for all participants, as well as for the team as a whole. The combination of clinically relevant scenarios for each sub-group should result in a meaningful and plausible overall scenario. In addition, both the tasks of the sub-groups as well as the resulting scenario for the complete team must have the potential to expose the patterns of within and between team communication and allow for events that are challenging as far as team performance is concerned.

Simulation technology presently available allows for clinically relevant and challenging scenarios for anaesthesiologists. By contrast, simulated surgical scenarios have not yet reached this standard. Though a large variety of surgical skill stations exist, their main purpose is to acquire basic manual skills. Once these skills are mastered further, rehearsal is of little, if any, perceived benefit. Thus, surgical skill stations do not allow for simulated scenarios sufficiently interesting to motivate experienced surgeons to participate in a complete operating room simulation. Simulation based on virtual reality may in the future provide scenarios that are sufficiently challenging. However, there is presently no scenario available that would meet our requirements. The main obstacles in building a simulator based on virtual reality are the computer power necessary to provide a complete surgical scenario with the appropriate sensory feedback.

The Need to Train Complete Teams

The operating team is composed of two distinct subgroups, the surgical team and the anaesthesia team. Most practitioners would probably agree that behaviour and the style of communication of their counterpart have a strong impact on their own behaviour and may even influence their own actions. This is in keeping with research performed in aviation showing that the behavioural pattern of captains has a strong impact on crew performance (Ginnett, 1993).

It is our strong belief that the ultimate goal in enhancing team performance in the operating room is the training of complete operating room teams. Although we acknowledge that sophisticated training programs based on simulator technology (e.g. crisis resource management for anaesthesiologists) are extremely valuable for training and teaching purposes, these programmes lack an important determinant of team performance: a surgeon performing surgery under plausible and clinically relevant conditions. Therefore, as far as enhancing team performance in the real operating room is concerned, these programmes have to be considered as 'part task training'. However, the above mentioned difficulties and problems encountered in our simulation programme with complete operating room teams may well indicate that part task training of sub-groups is, at least presently, the only achievable option.

The Role of Team Training in Professional Education

Team training in the simulator is embedded in a variety of activities related to human factors in the operating room. These include observations in real operating rooms, surveys on attitudes, seminars, research in the process of selecting anesthesia personnel, and an anonymous critical incident reporting system designed to be used on the internet (http://www.medana.unibas.ch/cirs/).

It is important to emphasise that team training cannot replace in-depth professional education. Instead technical proficiency of all personnel involved in patient care is a prerequisite for team training to be efficient and successful. Thus, our efforts in enhancing team performance should not jeopardise the quality of standard education. However, institutions and individuals have to recognise the need for education that goes beyond individual professional competence. As mentioned above, the ultimate goal in enhancing team performance should be the training of complete teams. Whether joint seminars of all groups of healthcare workers involved in the care of the patient in the operating room will find a broader acceptance than joint simulations remains to be seen.

REFERENCES

Brennan, T. A., L. L Leape, N. M. Laird *et al* (1991). Incidence of adverse events and negligence in hospitalized patients: results from the Harvard Medical Practice Study I. *New England Journal of Medicine*, **324**, 370-376.

Cooper, J. B., R. S. Newbower, C. D. Long, and B. J. McPeek (1978). Preventable anesthesia mishaps-a study of human factors. *Anesthesiology*, **49**, 399-406.

Cullen, D. J., B. J. Sweitzer, D. W. Bates, E. Burdick, A. Edmondson and L. Leape (1997). Preventable adverse drug events in hospitalized patients: a comparative study of intensive care and general care units. *Crit. Care Med.*, **25**, 1289-1297.

Donchin, Y., D. Gopher, M. Olin, Y. Badihi, M. Biesky, C. L. Sprung, R. Pizov and S. Cotev (1995) A look into the nature and causes of human errors in the intensive care unit. *Crit Care Med*, **2**, 294-300.

Ginnett, R.C. (1993). Crews as groups: their formation and leadership. In: *Cockpit Resource Management* (E. L. Wiener, B. G. Kanki and R. L. Helmreich, eds.), 71-98, Academic Press, San Diego.

Helmreich, R. L. and H. C. Foushee (1993). Why crew resource management? empirical and theoretical bases of human factors training in aviation. In: *Cockpit Resource Management* (E. L. Wiener, B. G. Kanki and R. L. Helmreich, eds.), 3-45, Academic Press, San Diego.

Helmreich, R. L. and A. C. Merritt (1998). LINE/LOS check list. In: *Culture at work in aviation and medicine* (R. L. Helmreich and A. C. Merritt, eds.), 261-264. Ashgate Publishing, Hants.

Leape, L. L., T. A. Brennan, N. M. Laird, *et al* (1991). The nature of adverse events in hospitalized patients: results from the Harvard Medical Practice Study II. *New England Journal of Medicine,* **324**, 377-384.

Marsch, S., C. Schori, B. Sexton, D. Scheidegger and C. Harms (1999). Training complete operating room teams in the simulator enhances team performance in the real operating room. *Anesthesiology* (Suppl).

Perper, J. A. (1994). Life-threatening and fatal therapeutic misadventures. In: *Human error in medicine* (M. S. Bogner, ed.), 27-52, Lawrence Erlbaum Associates, Hillsdale, USA.

Sexton, B., S. Marsch, R. Helmreich, D. Betzendoerfer, T. Kocher, D. Scheidegger, and the TOMS team (1998a). Jumpseating in the operating room. In: *Simulators in anesthesiology education* (L. Henson and A. Lee, eds.). Plenum Press, New York

Sexton, B., S. Marsch, R. Helmreich, D. Betzendoerfer, T. Kocher, D. Scheidegger, and the TOMS team (1998b). Participant evaluation of team orientated medical simulation. In: *Simulators in anesthesiology education* (L. Henson and A. Lee, eds.). Plenum Press, New York.

Williamson, J. A., R. K. Webb, A. Sellen, et al (1993). Human failure: an analysis of 2000 incident reports. *Anaesthesia and Intensive Care,* **21**, 678-683.

CHAPTER 9

ORGANISATIONAL INTERFACES, RISK POTENTIALS AND QUALITY LOSSES IN NURSING: A MULTI-LEVEL APPROACH

André Büssing, Jürgen Glaser, Britta Herbig, Technical University Munich

SUMMARY

At first glance, 'risk and safety in medicine' seems to be associated with accidents, deficiencies in ergonomics and more or less concrete technical aspects of work design. From an organisational psychologist's perspective, risks are also related to poorly designed working systems and an insufficient level of system integration. The consequences of risk potentials are much more than damage and injury, they may be integrated within the broader concept of quality losses. Accordingly, risk potentials can be conceptualised as frictional losses at organisational interfaces between different social or technical subsystems respectively between different organisational levels, which will probably result in quality losses in the long run. Against the background of the 'Organisation-Activity-Individual-Approach', a theoretical concept which provides a methodology for multi-level analysis of work in organisations, the paper focuses on the relationships between organisational interfaces, risk potentials and quality losses at different levels of the hospital organisation with respect to

- disturbances (e.g. interruptions) within the nursing subsystem due to tayloristic forms of work organisation;
- disturbances (e.g. hindrances) at the interface between nursing tasks and technological performance conditions;
- disturbances (e.g. communication problems) at the interface between the nursing and medicine subsystems due to poor system-integration;
- disturbances (e.g. non-usability) at the interface between nursing process and technological, computer-assisted solutions.

Empirical evidence from several studies in different hospital systems provides practical illustrations and points to the substantial costs of badly designed working systems in hospitals.

INTRODUCTION

Looking at 'risk and safety in medicine', reports of patients severely injured or even killed due to professional blunder by doctors or nurses come to mind first. With regard to the increasing use of technology in hospitals, new accident scenarios emerge - for example, technical breakdowns during surgery or the application of wrong medication because of storage problems or usability problems in a clinical information system. All these scenarios only represent the tip of the iceberg; the problems that pave the way for such sometimes disastrous errors lie deeper or under the surface of the system. They are risk potentials that are not always recognised as such but that may nevertheless lead to very difficult and severe situations in the long run.

In this chapter we attempt to integrate these problems from a work and organisational psychology perspective within the concept of quality losses. Their origin lies in poorly designed working systems and/or in an insufficient level of system integration. Hospitals are complex organisations, composed of a variety of technical and social subsystems, which offer many different organisational interfaces. It is these organisational interfaces which are in danger of quality losses, especially frictional losses.

In the following we refer to the term 'interface' as a point of contact between different organisational subsystems or members thereof. This may sometimes appear as mere interactions but rather it is the collision of sometimes conflicting subgoals due to the membership of the interacting persons in different subgroups (see below). Since the analysis of such risk potentials has to take many different levels into account, the 'Organisation-Activity-Individual-Approach' (Büssing, 1990, 1992) will be outlined in the next section. This is a theoretical framework which provides a multi-level analysis for work in organisations and which consequently allows a more specific consideration of potential quality losses at different organisational interfaces.

THE ORGANISATION-ACTIVITY-INDIVIDUAL-(OTI)-APPROACH

Most quality losses and risk potentials surface in the activities of the members of an organisation. As these activities are closely linked to the organisation on one side and the individual on the other side they are the culmination point of problems from all levels of a complex organisation. According to the Organisation-Activity-Individual-Approach, activity[1] in the working context is related to the organisation's basic conditions, that is the structure and the processes of the organisation, as it is also related to the individual who changes through the challenges and conditions of the activity. These relationships are not unidirectional, they transactionally work in both directions. The activity mediates the relationship between individual and organisation so that the dynamic interrelations between the different levels of an organisation are systematically taken into consideration. In detail, the different transitions can be characterised as follows:

- The transition between the individual and its activity comprises all processes of starting and controlling an activity by the individual, i.e. the regulation of the activity through personal motives.
- The transition between activity and organisation consists of the influence of the activity on the organisational structure, i.e. objective results of the activity.
- The transition between organisation and activity reflects the retroactive effect of the organisational structure on the activity, i.e. the influence of the degree of formalisation on the cooperation between professions.
- The transition between activity and individual describes the (retro)active effect of the activity on the individual, i.e. the impact of the activity on the individual's development of competencies, motivation and psycho-physical health.

This concept (see figure 9.1) reflects a multi-level process between the organisation and the individual, incorporating dynamic and structural elements which are mediated by individuals' activity (for empirical analysis see Büssing, 1992). At the organisational level there might be a change in the structure of a hospital. For instance, the implementation of a new nursing documentation system as one aspect of formalisation is performed in order to assess quality standards of nursing. At the level of the working tasks respectively working activities, this new documentation system might lead to additional demands. For example, nurses are obliged to document their measures accurately and in more detail than before. Under conditions of time pressure this may lead to a higher degree of strain experienced at the individual level. Higher levels of strain might in turn elicit risky behaviour by the nurse in order to get on with the work (activity level) and could reduce the quality of actual nursing work (organisational level).

---

[1] The term activity refers to the theoretical approach by Leont´ev and Vygotsky (e.g. Kozulin, 1986; Leont'ev, 1974) for an recent overview see Bedny & Meister, 1997) and its application in German work psychology by Hacker (1985, 1992) and Volpert (1974); for an overview see Frese and Zapf (1994).

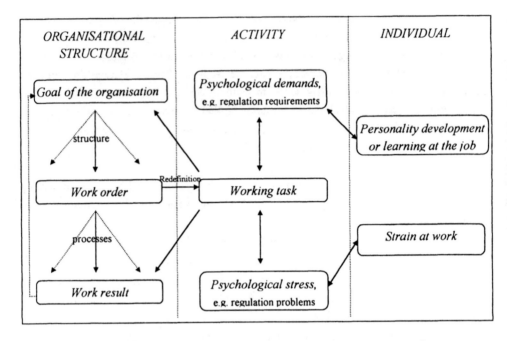

Figure 9.1   The Organisation-Activity-Individual (OTI) Approach[2]

The approach builds the background for the detailed analysis of each level of an organisation, as well as of the respective effects on other levels. From a methodological point of view, the existence and interdependence of different levels in organisations requires a level-specific diagnosis which has to fulfill two conditions. First, instruments have to be developed which are able to analyse and depict the specific characteristics of each level. Second, because multi-level analysis is not merely a mixture of different methods it has to be understood as a theory-based and integrated methodological strategy which reunites the level-specific results against a common conceptual background and therefore supports an integrated way of work and organisational design.

Analysis of working tasks, for example, requires observational methods since work behaviour is the focus of interest. Observations might give some hints, but do not sufficiently reveal the underlying mental processes of work regulation. Therefore, observations must be accompanied by interviews with the worker, dealing with the underlying psychological aspects of observed work behaviour. Furthermore, observations and interviews must be based on the same theoretical background and concepts – for example action regulation theory (see Frese and Zapf, 1994) and its concepts of regulation requirements and regulation problems - if the results are to be related to each other and should be integrated into a more comprehensive picture of work processes in hospitals' reality.

Using the OTI-Approach, the 'Work Analysis Instrument for Hospitals (Tätigkeits- und Arbeitsanalyseverfahren für das Krankenhaus - TAA-KH)' was developed by Büssing and Glaser (1999) in order to assess and evaluate the work in complex hospital organisations. The instrument which focuses on working conditions consists of different modules. A detailed analysis of the *organisation* level - the organisation diagnosis - is performed by means of interviews and analyses of documents in the expert rating version TAA-KH-O. At the level of nursing *activity* task analyses[3] are carried out on the wards by means of observation-interviews, i.e. complete shift observations by outside experts with supplementary interviews, in order to assess regulation requirements, regulation problems, additional effort and risky actions in nursing tasks. By means of the self-rating version TAA-KH-S, a condition-related questionnaire which encompasses the most essential characteristics of complete activity, nursing tasks are further analysed with regard to demands, latitudes, resources and stressors. Furthermore, on the *individual* level person-related questionnaires are administered assessing the individual's attitude towards work as well as psychophysiological health and health-related behaviour of the individual workers.

The 'Work Analysis Instrument for Hospitals (TAA-KH)' is conceptualised as a methodological multi-level and multi-method approach for specific analyses of working conditions at each level of the hospital organisation as well as for an integration of results at different levels against a common theoretical background. Therefore, it explicitly points at interfaces and offers the opportunity to inspect these interfaces between subsystems of the hospital organisation with respect to risk potentials and quality losses. In examining those interfaces from different viewpoints - from the organisational level, from the perspective of working tasks and task characteristics as well as from the individual's perspective - the validity of empirical results is substantially enhanced and the complex reality of a working system more adequately understood.

Interfaces as a Result of Work Organisation Within or Between Subsystems

Interfaces between different subsystems are outcomes of the process of dividing labour within the organisation. Division of labour can be performed in different ways and with different goals. First, basic determinants of work organisation are introduced before certain problems at different system interfaces, that are commonly due to the poorly designed architecture of working systems, will be examined. Looking at different forms of work organisation within the nursing subsystem seems to be a suitable approach for pointing out the principles and effects of the division of labour on the structure of working tasks and on the degree of system integration.

---

[2]   The illustration is taken from Glaser (1997).

[3]   The term task analysis refers to a specific method of data collection. Psychological relevant characteristics of working tasks like aspects of job demands and work load are investigated by means of expert ratings in the course of shift observations and interviews.

The traditional organisation of hospitals in Germany is based on a hierarchical structure with clear divisions and subordination relationships. On the ward this hierarchical organisation is transformed into a functional or tayloristic division of labour. In functional nursing the ward nurse coordinates the work processes on the ward by assigning working functions, or tasks, to certain nurses. The nurses perform the working functions in so-called 'rounds'. Within one round all patients on the ward are, for example, supplied with medication, which might have been prepared by a different nurse during the preceding night. Here, nursing is functional, or task-oriented, where each task is carried out by a different nurse, each having no detailed overview of the process as a whole. Behind this division of labour stands the one-sided traditional notion that only a technical determined specialisation of nursing leads to a maximum of quality and that not everybody can and should do everything (Büssing, 1997). This view of organising work has serious implications for nursing; nursing tasks are often incomplete since planning or controlling functions are often allocated by other persons or professions (e.g. ward nurse, doctor). Moreover, nursing is segmented into several different functions concerning mostly the medical state of the patient. Therefore, possible interactions between 'parts' of the patient, e.g. social situation, medical and psychological state, 'parts' of the nurse, e.g. workload, work satisfaction, and interaction in the relationship of both are at best underestimated, in the worst case neglected or even denied. Possible outcomes of these problems are summarised within the OTI approach in figure 9.3 (page 170).

Over the last couple of years this functional care has been the focus of criticism (e.g. Elkeles, 1994). Besides economic concepts that include the so-called human capital (qualification, motivation, health of the workers) and that refute the idea of economic advantages through functional nursing, other important points regarding quality losses and risk potentials are made. They apply to nurses working in functional care as well as to their patients. First of all, Elkeles (1994) demonstrated disadvantages in the time economy, i.e. nurses have to make unnecessary journeys, there are process inherent delays and increasing coordination requirements. Moreover, higher error rates due to vague arrangements or deficient coordination occurred in wards with a tayloristic work organisation. And, regarding the individual, a decrease in motivation and work satisfaction could be observed, so that these results clearly hint at risk potentials within the nursing subsystem.

Quality losses are also to be expected in the area of patient orientation (e.g. Feuerstein and Badura, 1991). In functional nursing the needs of the patient are secondary to the requirements of the nursing work organisation. The different rounds for different tasks and therefore the continuous changing intertwined with a high turnover rate of nurses due to stress and dissatisfaction hinders the development of trustful relationships between patient and nurse. Patient orientation does not just mean that patients should become clients and nursing should become a service. Rather, patient orientation expresses that the patient is taken seriously not only in his role as a patient but also with his living conditions, his relationships and his social environment. The patient is no longer object but subject; he becomes a partner in the nursing process. To some extent functional nursing with its division of labour, rationalistic structures, and formalised processes interferes with the kind of relationship between patient and nurse necessary for the realisation of patient orientation. Consequently, the lack of patient orientation due to a dysfunctional work organisation (Elkeles, 1994) mirrors quality losses that may even lead to prolonged hospital stays and more complications (Fagin, 1982a/b).

An extensively discussed alternative to functional nursing is the concept of holistic nursing (for details see Büssing, 1997; Glaser and Büssing, 1996a). The psychological concept of complete activity ('Konzept der vollständigen Tätigkeit') meets the demand for a holistic nursing from the nurses' perspective (e.g. Büssing, 1992; Hacker, 1985). This concept states that work activities can unfold their health and personality enhancing potential only if several conditions are met. Among these conditions one finds the variety of requirements, possibility for social interaction, opportunities for learning and development, and meaningfulness of tasks. The psychological concept of complete activity in nursing can at least lessen the individual problems discussed for functional, or task-oriented, nursing. Within the 'Organisation-Activity-Individual-Approach', strain and stress at work and the risk potentials related to them can be supplanted by personality development and opportunities for learning. An evaluation study on the development of a holistic nursing system underlines the fruitful effects of complete task structures in nursing. The results give evidence for a better degree of system-integration between nursing and other organisational subsystems as well as for the nursing system itself (Büssing *et al.*, 1997a).

The following sections of the chapter focus on risk potentials and quality losses at three specific interfaces within the hospital system due to certain forms of work organisation. *First*, we look at the frictions within the nursing system. Results and examples used to illustrate these frictions derive from a series of studies collected over time (4 points of measurement), which were performed in order to evaluate the process of developing the nursing system in a general hospital from functional to holistic nursing within the period of 1994-1997. *Second*, we examine the cooperation at the interface between nursing system and medical subsystems. Data provided for illustration was once again collected within the longitudinal study mentioned previously. *Third*, results from another evaluation study of a nursing information system performed during the period of 1996-1997 in our laboratory are presented; they can illustrate potential risks and benefits at the interface between the social and technical subsystem.

The Interface between Nursing Tasks and Technological Performance Conditions

Frictions within the nursing subsystem can be conceptualised as discrepancies between nursing tasks and performance conditions as summarised in figure 9.3 (page 170). According to the concept of regulation problems respectively the broader concept of contradictory demands (e.g. Glaser and Büssing, 1996b; Leitner *et al.*, 1987; Moldaschl, 1991), contradictions between task and technological performance conditions (Perrow, 1965) lead to additional effort or risky action and therefore may cause risk potentials and quality losses.

Within the scope of a longitudinal study, a project aiming at the implementation of a holistic nursing system was evaluated from a work and organisational psychology perspective. Four wards of a general hospital participating in the project were investigated by means of the 'Work Analysis Instrument for Hospitals' [TAA-KH] as well as by questionnaires for analysing attitudes, well-being and behaviour of the nurses over a period of three years at four points of measurement. Comparisons between 'project wards', all other wards of the hospital and the wards of two other structurally comparable general hospitals were carried out at the start (T1) and at the end of the project (T4). Altogether 64 whole shift observations and 96 interviews with nurses at 32 wards, 19 interviews with the hospital managers and other experts of the organisation were performed, and questionnaires to a representative sample of 482 nurses in the three hospitals at T1 were administered. At T4 a representative sample of 474 nurses could be reached by questionnaire, and 56 whole shift observations and 84 interviews with nurses at 28 wards as well as 19 interviews with hospital managers and experts were performed. Analyses of documents and statistics were carried out in order to complete the fundament of the organisational diagnosis. Using the TAA-KH several kinds of regulation problems in the daily routine of nurses could be identified (Büssing *et al.*, 1997b) (see examples in table 9.1).

On the side of impediments, informational and motorical problems were differentiated. Informational problems in nursing exist if necessary information for certain tasks is not available, not recognisable, not clear or ambiguous, if it is wrong, erroneous or incomplete, or if the necessary information is not available in time or could not be passed on. Regarding technology this kind of complication is likely to occur in the implementation phase of hospital or care information systems, as there might be problems with the transfer and actualisation of data or the timely recording of relevant information (e.g. problem of recording data at the bedside and transferring them to the main terminal). The risk potential of these informational problems are obvious: The danger of errors occurring because important or even vital information about a patient is not available is great, especially on wards where high rates of information have to be processed. Motorical problems as another kind of possible impediment in nursing refer to hindrances in movement and in the use of working materials. Old or badly designed rooms, devices and working materials must be compensated by additional effort by the nurses, which will lead to quality losses.

TABLE 9.1

Aspects of regulation problems within the nursing subsystem and their consequences in
additional effort and risky actions

Regulation problems	Examples	Consequences (additional effort/risky action)
Informational impediments	Unreadable hand-writing, missing patient data	Trying to reach responsible persons (usually doctors); risk of mistakes, e.g. wrong medicine orders, wrong diagnosis concerning acute problems
Motorical impediments	Small patient rooms, lack of tools for lifting patients	Time-consuming removal of furniture; Danger of injuring oneself, damage of intervertebral discs
Interruptions due to persons	Telephone calls during patient care	Resumption or new beginning of nursing activities; danger to forget important measures; quality losses and reduced degree of patient orientation
Interruptions due to malfunction	Flaws in equipment	Walk to other wards in order to borrow equipment or devices; Danger to patient's life in case of vital treatment (e.g. administering oxygen, monitoring vital signs)
Interruptions due to blockades	Unavailable elevators	Waiting in front of the elevator; danger in case of emergency removal to ICU or patient transport from surgery

Interruptions as another form of regulation problems can be due to people, malfunctions, and
blockades. The interruptions and their consequences will be discussed in the context of the
interface between medical and nursing subsystem. Interruptions in the continuity of work
processes could be caused not only by physicians but also by interruptions from the
administrative subsystem or from the relatives of patients. Malfunctions of devices are
another possible source of interruptions in the nursing process. Necessary actions have to
wait until the devices are repaired or a substitute has been found. In routine work this may
only lead to additional demands on the nurse but in case of an emergency such malfunctions
have a high inherent risk potential, e.g. a dysfunctional oxygen apparatus. The same problems
hold for blockades, i.e. the nurses have to wait in order to carry on with their tasks (e.g.

waiting for elevators). This again may lead to quality losses in the routine work but in an emergency risky situations may follow due to blockades (for details about the frequency of the occurrence of regulation hindrances see Büssing *et al.*, 1997b; Glaser, 1997).

The contradictory demands that derive from regulation problems are closely interrelated with necessary redefinitions of working tasks by the nurses. Breakdowns or malfunctions of technological conditions on the ward lead to the question of how to cope with the situation. Possible answers to this question range from a compensation of the problem through additional efforts to reactions of risky behavior both due to the pressure and strain experienced in the situation (see table 9.1). According to the empirical results from task analyses on 32 wards, additional effort due to regulation problems reaches up to 120 minutes in some wards, nearly half of it caused by interruptions by people (Glaser, 1997). Moreover, during the shift observations situations could be registered in which quality losses and risky action occur due to technical deficiencies, interruptions, time pressure etc. For example, there is no opportunity to manage the situation if a nurse has to wait for the elevator in case of an emergency requiring the fast transfer of a patient to the ICU. In situations of high time pressure, certain tasks might be carried out at speed, some only partially and some perhaps not at all, for instance, controlling medicine before giving it to the patients or documenting patient-related observations. The likelihood of administering the wrong medicine or of failing to note an important reaction of a patient might be rather low, but if it should occur the consequences could be lethal.

The Interface between Medical and Nursing Subsystems

The typical hospital structure usually consists of at least three different subsystems - the administrative subsystem, the medical and the nursing subsystem. To fulfill the goals of the organization and the working tasks within each of these subsystems a lot of communication and exchange has to take place at the interfaces between the subsystems (see, for example, Badura *et al.*, 1993; Winter, 1994). In particular, the medical and nursing subsystems need a strong integration in order to work efficiently and effectively not only for the sake of the patient but also to minimise stress and strain for the nurses, the doctors and other groups of professions concerned with patient care and treatment. Problems at this interface are very likely to result in quality losses which on one side are directly linked to disturbances in work processes and indirectly linked to errors due to psychological strain of the staff (see figure 9.3, page 170).

Büssing *et al.* (1996) examined interfaces between medical and nursing subsystems with respect to cooperation and communication. The analyses were performed on the data based on the first point of measurement (T1) in the longitudinal study, described above, which compared three hospitals over a period of three years. Cooperation and communication were evaluated according to the OTI-Approach from different perspectives and with different methods. Interviews with hospital managers provided a top-down perspective on the quality and the problems at the interface between the medical and nursing subsystems. By shift observations and interviews with nurses and doctors a complementary bottom-up perspective was taken which provides process-related and concrete aspects of cooperation and communication problems at the interfaces. In addition, 482 nurses assessed the quality of cooperation and communication within a questionnaire. Grounded Theory (Strauss and Corbin, 1996) was used as the basis for the analysis of the qualitative data. Contacts at the interfaces were coded according to preceding and intervening conditions, interactional strategies and their consequences.

The overall picture drawn by this study showed that the quality of interfaces between physicians and nursing colleagues was rated relatively negative, particularly when the inter-actions were intensive and frequent. The analysis also revealed that there were more conflicts in social aspects and cooperation concerning planning than concerning execution. This means that, due to hierarchical structures and a lack of communication, the planning of work processes in the medical subsystem was not coordinated with work processes in the nursing subsystem. For instance, the doctors' rounds were fixed according to the time pressures of the physicians, whereas the nurses had to interrupt their respective work for these rounds.

Inadequate understanding of working processes, including time restriction in other subsystems, little communication for planning and tuning cooperative processes, individualistic perspectives and interests in different hierarchical structures as well as interpersonal problems impede the improvement of such quality losses.

Typical situations of interface problems between nursing and medicine were:

- Doctors' rounds were seldom scheduled, consequently causing daily interruptions in nursing.
- Doctors were using the documentation system while the nurses needed to use it.
- Medical orders were made 'en passant', running the risk of misunderstandings and oblivion.
- Unregulated allocation of responsibilities between nurses and doctors (e.g. injections, medication on demand).
- Lack of information and insight with regard to each other's work organisation.
- Availability of doctors etc.

The following statements from different interviews might illustrate some of these problems: *"You can ask whom you want, but nobody knows it"* (a doctor's view about the responsibility of nurses for certain patients within a holistic nursing system); *"Structures are often used as an excuse for individual incompetence"* (example for an individualistic explanation pattern for quality losses at the interface); *"We get along very well and don't want to have problems with each other, but I think that the others can't manage the requirements either"* (explanation of quality losses due to time pressure and too high demands for all subsystems).

With regard to the risk potentials, the study described shows a pressing problem at the interface between medical and nursing subsystem grounded in poor system integration as illustrated in figure 9.1 (see page 158). The example of the "doctors' rounds problem" suggests at least short term quality losses and risk potentials: The interruption of nursing processes may interfere with the completing of tasks that are important for the patient, leading at best to dissatisfaction and, in the worst case, to risky behaviour due to the fact that the nurse wants to meet all requirements in the situation. In the long run, this risk potential might increase as the steady strain along the interface may exhaust the resources of the nurses.

The Interface between Nursing Process and Technological, Computer-Assisted Solutions

Over recent years more and more hospitals in Germany have implemented hospital information systems (HIS) to handle the growing amount of data that has to be processed (e.g. Büssing and Herbig, 1998a/b). The prevailing situation in the development of HIS shows that they are most often not homogenous or closed but a structure of different systems which are implemented at different times (e.g. Winter and Haux, 1995). Until now, there has been no commonly accepted definition of HIS, so we have adopted the following description: HIS is the partial system within hospitals that conducts computer-supported information processing and storage. Its concrete tasks include the disposition of patient information, information on diseases, medication as well as quality of treatment and costs. An effectively working HIS needs at least three different components (e.g. Hannan, 1991): the *hospital management system* for support of administrative activities as well as non-medical supply and technics, e.g. maintenance and repairs; the *clinical information system* including support of all medical and care activities as well as aspects of medical supply; and the *electronic patient record* at the centre of the clinical information system in which all patient-related data are stored, preferably in a relational database. In order for a HIS to work effectively and efficiently, the interfaces between these components need to be functioning or else communication between different hospital areas will not be possible. Besides this technical necessity one of the biggest challenges is the integration of very different subsystems and the consideration of the needs of each subgroup. The usability of such a HIS is of utmost importance not only for its acceptance, but also for error- and risk-free handling.

The structure of HIS described above shows the central position of the clinical information system with the electronic patient record at its core. Since the highest accumulation of data occurs on the ward as a 'turntable' of all patient-related information, a usability study of the care information system PIK ('Pflegedienst im Krankenhaus') will be presented and possible disturbances at the interface between task (i.e. nursing process) and the programme discussed (Büssing and Herbig, 1998c).

As the programme PIK[4] was designed to support nursing in hospitals, the following questions were addressed in a laboratory study: How do potential users deal intuitively with the programme? What problems and errors may occur during working with the programme? And how does the system support the nursing process? A sample of 11 nurses and nursing students were asked to deal with different modules of the system (nursing standards and care planning), while verbal protocols (Ericsson and Simon, 1993) were recorded and occurring errors rated into a taxonomy based on German action regulation theory (e.g. Zapf, 1991). This kind of taxonomy has the concrete advantage that one can state the stage of action regulation in which the error occurs. This allows not only recommendations for user training but also the detection of system inherent risk potentials. Zapf (1991) differentiates three different kinds of errors: 'inefficient action', 'problems in functioning' and 'problems in using', whereby inefficient action is separated from manifest errors because goal attainment is possible with inefficient action. Problems in functioning can be seen as a mismatch between task and computer, and problems in using that are in the center of the taxonomy show the mismatch between user and system on different stages of the action regulation.

The 'problems in using' the system are vertically divided in the different stages of action regulation (see table 9.2) - the planning phase, i.e. goal setting and designing of a plan for reaching the goal, the monitoring phase, i.e. the supervision of plan execution whereby plan and subplans must be remembered, and the feedback phase, i.e. evaluating if the goal is reached. Furthermore, a horizontal division into different levels of regulation takes place. At the level of intellectual regulation one find conscious analysis and synthesis processes for the regulation of complex activities for which no ready pattern of activity exist. The level of flexible activity pattern consists of already existing basic pattern for the required activity that have to be adapted for the situation. Processes at this level are conscious, they are not automated but already mastered. At the sensomotor level highly automated activities take place. Because they are no longer conscious, no planning or feedback loops are detectable. This matrix of level and stages leads to eight different kinds of 'errors in using' that were recorded by the experimenter during the execution of a task by the test persons, for example:

- *Knowledge error*: A programme is unknown to a person and therefore errors occur.
- *Thought errors*: While planning an action, important features of the programme are not taken into account.
- *Noticing/ Forgetting error*: While executing a task an earlier planned step is forgotten.
- *Judgement error*: A system feedback is misinterpreted.
- *Habitual error*: An already known path of action is used although it is wrong.
- *Omission error*: Changes have not been saved.
- *Recognition error*: The overview over a mask is lost although it is known to the person.
- *Movement error*: Wrong double clicking.

---

[4] For a detailed description of the programme and its different modules see Wolfrum, Schneider & Herbig, 1997.

TABLE 9.2

Error Taxonomy adapted from Zapf (1991)

Problems in functioning			
Action Blockade	System blockades the reaching of goals		
Action Repetition	Parts of the work get lost and must be repeated		
Action Interruption	Working process is interrupted and can be continued only after waiting		
Action Roundabout	Functional problem must be compensated by additional effort		
Problems in using			
Regulation Basis	Knowledge Error		
Regulation Level	Process stages		
	Goals/Planning	**Memory/Monitoring**	**Feedback**
Intellectual regulation level	Thought error	Noticing/Forgetting error	Judgment error
Level of flexible action patterns	Habitual error	Omission error	Recognition error
Sensomotor regulation level	Movement error		
Roundabouts			
Inefficiency due to habit			
Inefficiency due to insufficient knowledge			

While the actual use of the programme proved to be quite easy even for novices in the area of electronic data processing, the conceptual structuring of the system and the nursing data master file caused difficulties for the participants (as seen in the many errors on the intellectual regulation level in working with the nursing standards, figure 9.2). These difficulties mainly stemmed from problems of generating a clear mental picture of the system and the consequences of ones' actions, i.e. due to the lack of system feedback the test persons got lost and felt irritated while trying to complete an activity with the system. This was seen in the error rate on the feedback stage in working with the care planning module. Regarding the question of quality losses and risk potentials, the relevance of such results is easy to see. The importance of correct, complete and timely information in nursing and medicine has already been discussed and the results of this study show two factors that may lead to disturbances in the flow of information. On one side, problems of orientation within the program lead to confusion regarding the question if the planned goal is reached. This in turn may cause the termination of an action although the goal was not reached, thus, leading to the loss of information. On the other hand lacking usability leads to frustration and a reluctance to use the system, thereby disturbing the necessary data flow and leading once again to quality losses or even risky situations when vital information is not available.

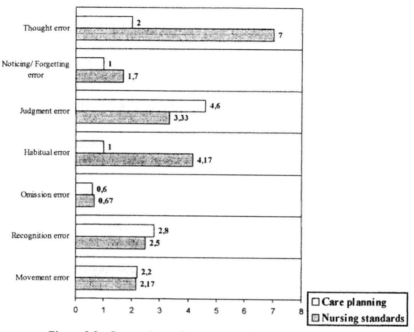

Figure 9.2   Comparison of error means between two modules of the system PIK

Another important result of this kind of research refers to the kind of work organisation. Although the program PIK is designed for the support of holistic nursing it may as well become a tool for functional nursing. The concept 'Technology as an option' (e.g. Ulich, 1998) proposes that the crucial point is not the software itself but the underlying concept of work design. Experiences from industry show that existing organisational concepts are reinforced by the implementation of new technologies. As a consequence, a care information system for the support of holistic nursing will only fulfill its purpose if holistic nursing is already practiced or explicit efforts are undertaken to implement such a work design. EDP-plans without such a fundamental decision serve pure technology design and may reinforce existing unfavorable organisational structures and their already discussed risk potentials. With respect to the socio-technical match between task, user, and system the interface between computer-assisted solutions and nursing tasks is a good example for the necessity of multi-level analysis of risk potentials and quality losses. The organisational goal of efficient and error-free data processing encloses all subsystems; this bearing the risk with each electronic interface of system problems that lead to the loss or incompleteness of data thus to information hindrances that must be compensated by the individual. A mismatch between the user and the system may as well lead to problems in the flow of information and last but not least the system may enhance unfavorable work structures that also can cause risky behaviour and quality losses in nursing. Each of these levels is connected via several feedback loops with the other levels so that errors on one level may spread through the whole organisation.

OUTLOOK

The chapter started with scenarios of risky situations in hospitals, proposing that they are only the peak of more common problems that may evolve to dangerous situations. Four different but intertwined problems at the interface between different social or technical subsystems and in the work organisation within subsystems were presented to demonstrate disturbances that may lead to quality losses and risk potentials in nursing (for a summary and integration in the OTI approach see figure 9.3). A crucial question remains to be answered: How can these quality losses and risk potentials be prevented or at least minimised?

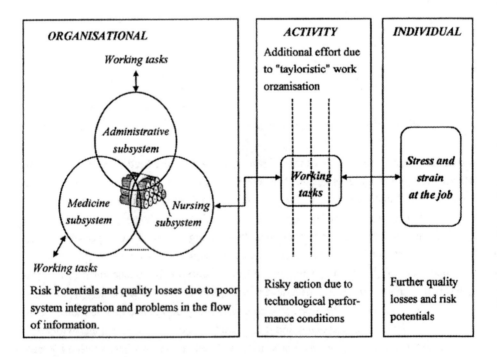

Figure 9.3 Quality losses and risk potentials in the Organisation-Activity-Individual-Approach

According to the multi-level approach, the answer has different facets. First of all, each level or subsystem itself has to be reorganized in such a way that the discussed problems are not likely to occur. Therefore, detailed analysis of the goals, structure and working processes, as well as the disturbances within a system, have to take place. The TAA-KH is an instrument for analysis in the nursing subsystem (Büssing and Glaser, 1999). Advice for reorganisation should be based on such an extensive analysis. For example, the implementation of holistic nursing systems proved to be a fruitful approach for organisational development in hospitals.

The results of the evaluation study concerning costs and benefits of developing a nursing system from functional to holistic nurses showed that the reorganisation of nursing processes not only decreased work load (e.g. regulation obstacles due to interruptions) to a considerably degree (statistically significant changes over four times of measurement) and increased the quality of working life (e.g. job satisfaction of nurses), but also improved the interface between nurses and patients regarding the quality of service (for details see Büssing *et al.*, 1997a).

The same holds for other social or technological subsystems. For example, computer-assisted information systems should be developed according to a detailed requirements definition (e.g. Ball *et al.*, 1995) again based in extensive analysis of the situation and subsequent goals. Here the qualification of the staff is of special interest. The implementation of computer-aided information and documentation systems often fails due to a lack of user acceptance, especially those who are insufficiently involved in the choice and implementation of such systems and/or who are not properly instructed in the use of the system. Moreover, regarding computer-aided care planning, nurses in German hospitals are still not qualified enough to perform individual and planned care in the sense of the nursing process model. Such deficiencies in qualification must be addressed before the implementation of computer-aided solutions. Failing this, such systems represent a clear overstrain for the nursing staff.

More interesting and less clear is the answer to the question of the circumvention of interface problems. An often mentioned probate way of organisational design is the reduction of interfaces (e.g. Badura *et al.*, 1993) and hierarchy levels for optimising organisational processes. Regarding the interface between the nursing and medicine subsystem and the patients this seems to be the obvious solution since patient orientation and the development of a trustful relationship depends on the constancy of the care giver. Alternatively, Büssing *et al.* (1996) draw another conclusion for the interfaces between nursing and medical subsystem - not the reduction of interfaces but the enlargement can be a helpful measure to prevent quality losses. A stronger linkage between the different professional groups may help to preserve and to use the existing experience and knowledge. Or, as Endres and Wehner (1995) stated, the improvement of organisational processes can make additional communication and forms of integration a necessity. Here the subsystems are not only seen as organisational, formal units but as social groups consisting of individuals with their own redefinition of goals and tasks that are to be modeled, i.e. all three levels of the 'Organisation-Activity-Individual-Approach' have to be taken into account. A possibility for the improvement of organisational interfaces can be interdisciplinary work groups that analyse and evaluate weak points, e.g. by means of standardised methods like the TAA-KH, and - in the sense of quality circles - work out solutions for the improvement of these problematic points.

REFERENCES

Badura, B., G. Feuerstein and T. Schott, (eds.) (1993). *System Krankenhaus. Arbeit, Technik und Patientenorientierung* [System Hospital. Work, technology, and patient orientation]. Weinheim: Juventa.

Ball, M. J., K. J. Hannah, S. K Newbold and J. V. Douglas, (eds.) (1995). *Nursing Informatics. Where caring and technology meet.* New York: Springer.

Bedny, G. and D. Meister (1997). *The Russian theory of activity: Current applications to design and learning.* Erlbaum, Mahwah, NJ

Büssing, A. (1990). Die Interaktion der Ebenen als Problem komplexer Organisationen [The interaction of levels as a problem of complex organizations]. In: *Vom Umgang mit Komplexität in Organisationen* [About dealing with complexity in organizations] (R. Fisch and M. Boos, eds.), pp. 63-94. Universitätsverlag, Konstanz

Büssing, A. (1992). *Organisationsstruktur, Tätigkeit und Individuum* [Organizational structure, activity and the individual]. Huber, Bern.

Büssing, A. (1997). Neue Entwicklungen in der Krankenpflege. Von der funktionalen zur ganzheitlichen Pflege [New developments in nursing. From functional to holistic nursing]. In: *Von der funktionalen zur ganzheitlichen Krankenpflege. Reorganisation von Dienstleistungsprozessen im Krankenhaus* [From functional to holistic nursing. Reorganisation of service processes in hospitals] (A. Büssing, ed.), pp. 15-48. Verlag für Angewandte Psychologie, Göttingen.

Büssing, A., M. Barkhausen and J. Glaser (1996). Schnittstellen im Krankenhaus. Analyse aus der Sicht des Pflegedienstes am Beispiel von Kooperation und Kommunikation. [Interfaces in the hospital. Analysis from the nursing perspective with the examples cooperation and communication]. *Zeitschrift für Arbeitswissenschaft,* **50** (3), 129-138.

Büssing, A., M. Barkhausen, J. Glaser and S. Schmitt. (1997a). Evaluation der Einführung eines ganzheitlichen Pflegesystems [Evaluation of the implementation of a holistic nursing system] (Report Nr. 41). Technische Universität, Lehrstuhl für Psychologie, München.

Büssing, A., M. Barkhausen, J. Glaser and S. Schmitt (1997b). Psychischer Streß und Burnout in der Krankenpflege. Ergebnisse im Längsschnitt [Psychological stress and burnout in nursing. A longitudinal study] (Report Nr. 37). Technische Universität, Lehrstuhl für Psychologie, München.

Büssing, A. and J. Glaser (1999). *Das Tätigkeits- und Analyseverfahren für das Krankenhaus - Selbstbeobachtungsversion (TAA-KH-S)* [Work Analysis Instrument for Hospitals - selfrating-version]. Hogrefe, Göttingen.

Büssing, A. and B. Herbig (1998a). Recent developments of Care Information Systems in Germany. *Computers in Nursing,* **16**, 307-310.

Büssing, A. and B. Herbig (1998b). The challenges of a Care Information System reflecting holistic nursing care. *Computers in Nursing,* **16**, 311-317.

Büssing, A. and B. Herbig (1998c). Das Pflegeinformationssystem PIK: Eine arbeitspsychologische Exploration zur Usability [The care information system PIK: A work psychological exploration of usability]. *Zeitschrift für Arbeitswissenschaft,52,* 240-249.

Elkeles, T. (1994). *Arbeitsorganisation in der Krankenpflege. Zur Kritik der Funktionspflege.* [Work organization in nursing. Critique of functional care]. Mabuse-Verlag, Frankfurt.

Endres, E. and T. Wehner (1995). Störungen zwischenbetrieblicher Kommunikation [Disturbances in interorganisational communication]. In: *Managementforschung 5. Empirische Studien* [Management research 5. Empirical studies] (G. Schreyögg and J. Sydow, eds.), pp. 1-45. De Gruyter, Berlin.

Ericsson, K. A. and H. A. Simon (1993). *Protocol Analysis - Verbal Reports as Data.* Bradford, Cambridge.

Fagin, C. M. (1982a). Nursing as an alternative to high-cost-care. *American Journal of Nursing,* **82** (1), 56-60.

Fagin, C. M. (1982b). The economic value of nursing research. *American Journal of Nursing,* **82** (12), 1844-1849.

Feuerstein, G. and B. Badura (1991). *Patientenorientierung durch Gesundheitsförderung im Krankenhaus* [Patient orientation through health promotion in the hospital]. Hans Böckler Stiftung, Düsseldorf.

Frese, M. and D. Zapf (1994). Action as the core of work psychology: A German approach. In: *Handbook of industrial and organizational psychology Vol. 4* (H. C. Triandis, M. D. Dunnette and L. M. Hough, eds.), pp. 271-340. Consulting Psychologists Press, Palo Alto, Cal.

Glaser, J. (1997). *Aufgabenanalysen in der Krankenpflege. Eine arbeitspsychologische Analyse und Bewertung pflegerischer Aufgaben* [Task analysis in nursing. A work psychological analysis and evaluation of nursing activities]. Waxmann, Münster.

Glaser, J. and A. Büssing (1996a). Ganzheitliche Pflege: Präzisierung und Umsetzungschancen [Holistic nursing: Specification and chances for realization]. *Pflege,* **9,** 221-232.

Glaser, J. and A. Büssing (1996b). Widersprüchliche Anforderungen in der Arbeitstätigkeit, Zusatzaufwand und psychischer Streß. Konzepte und Überprüfung eines Vermittlungsmodells [Contradictory demands in work activity, additional effort and psychological stress. Concept and investigation of a mediating model]. *Zeitschrift für Arbeits- und Organisationspsychologie,* **40** (2), 87-91.

Hacker, W. (1985). Activity - A fruitful concept in industrial psychology. In: *Goal directed behavior: The concept of action in psychology* (M. Frese and J. Sabini, eds.), pp. 262-284). Erlbaum, Hillsdale, NJ.

Hacker, W. (1992). Action regulation theory and occupational psychology, Review of German empirical research since 1987. *German Journal of Psychology,* **18,** 91-120.

Hannan T. (1991). Medical informatics - an Australian perspective. *Australian and New Zealand Journal of Medicine*, **21**, 363-378.

Kozulin, A. (1986). The concept of activity in Sovjet psychology. Vygotsky, his disciples and critics. *American Psychologist*, **41**, 264-274.

Leitner, K., W. Volpert, B. Greiner, W. G. Weber and K. Hennes (1987). *Analyse psychischer Belastungen in der Arbeit. Das RHIA-Verfahren. Handbuch* [Analysis of psychological strain at work. The RHIA-procedure. Handbook]. Verlag TÜV Rheinland, Köln.

Leont'ev, A. N. (1974). The problem of activity in psychology. *Soviet Psychology*, (Winter), 4-33.

Moldaschl, M. (1991). *Frauenarbeit oder Facharbeit?* [Women work or skilled work?] a.M. Campus, Frankfurt.

Perrow, C. (1965). Hospitals: Technology, structure, and goals. In: *Handbook of Organizations* (G. March, ed.), pp. 910-971. Rand Mc. Nally, Chicago.

Strauss, A. and J. Corbin (1996). *Grounded Theory: Grundlagen qualitativer Sozialforschung* [Grounded Theory: Foundations of qualitative social research]. PVU, Weinheim.

Ulich, E. (1998). *Arbeitspsychologie* [Work psychology], 4th ed. Stuttgart: Schäffer-Poeschel.

Volpert, W. (1974). Handlungsstrukturanalyse [Structural analysis of action]. Pahl-Rugenstein, Köln.

Winter A. and R. Haux (1995). A Three-Level Graph-Based Model for the Management of Hospital Information Systems. *Methods of Information in Medicine*, **34**, 378-396.

Winter, C. (1994). Auswirkungen des EDV-Einsatzes auf das soziale System 'Krankenhaus' [Consequences of EDP on the social system „hospital"]. *Zeitschrift für Gesundheitswissenschaften*, **2** (4), 315-323.

Wolfrum, R. B. Schneider and B. Herbig (1997). Informations und Kommunikationssysteme im Krankenhaus und neue Formen der Arbeitsorganisation in der Pflege [Information-and communication technologies in hospitals and new forms of work organization in nursing]. In: *Von der funktionalen zur ganzheitlichen Pflege. Reorganisation von Dienstleistungsprozessen im Krankenhaus* [From functional to holistic nursing. Reorganisation of service processes in hospitals], (A. Büssing ed.), pp. 135-161. Hogrefe, Göttingen.

Zapf, D. (1991). Taxonomie von Handlungsfehlern bei der Computerarbeit [Taxonomy of action errors in computer work]. In: *Fehler bei der Arbeit mit dem Computer. Ergebnisse von Beobachtungen und Befragungen im Bürobereich* [Errors in the work with computers. Results of observations and interviews in offices] (M. Frese and D. Zapf, eds.), pp. 32-46. Huber, Bern.

CHAPTER 10

CONTROLLING THE RISKS OF MECHANICAL HEART VALVE FAILURE USING PRODUCT LIFE CYCLE-BASED SAFETY MANAGEMENT

Manon Cromheecke, Floor Koornneef, Geerda van Gaalen, Bas de Mol
Delft University of Technology and Department of Cardio-thoracic Surgery, Academic Medical Centre of the University of Amsterdam, The Netherlands

INTRODUCTION

Biomedical implants and devices are one of the most important developments of the biomedical industrial progress in modern healthcare (Starr, 1986). Highly skilled professionals and stringent manufacturing processes are essential to ensure quality and long-term performance, but assessing the safety and risk of failure are equally important. However, analyses of safety are usually focused on technical qualities, neglecting problems with the implant/carrier interface, limitations in durability, and the high expectations of both clinicians and patients. In the near future, we are likely to see the development and use of so-called smart devices, which are programmable in a similar way to pacemakers for cardiac stimulation, raising new and more complex safety issues (de Mol *et al.*, 1995; Black, 1996).

When the risk is lethal and the implant difficult to replace, risk control strategies are difficult to generate and to execute. Structural failures of mechanical heart valves pose great challenges for risk control (de Mol *et al.*, 1994, 1995). Other frequent, disabling, and sometimes lethal, complications of a mechanical heart valve are bleeding and thromboembolism in the presence of the mandatory use of anticoagulant therapy. Recently, self-test kits in the form of a home-laboratory have become available for patients to keep the blood thinning well within the safe range. So, patients are now exposed to two devices: the valve and the blood thinning tester, both of which enhance survival but also introduce complexity and additional risk. The self-test named CoaguChek® has been used by over 15,000 patients so far and is currently under investigation by several groups. (Hasenkam *et al.*, 1997)

We studied the unprecedented number of mechanical heart valve failures of Björk-Shiley convexo-concave (BScc) mechanical heart valves, which were manufactured between 1979 and 1986. Failure of BScc valves has been reported for over 20 years, with the first fracture of this type reported in 1978. A poorly controlled design and manufacturing process have led to fatigue fractures, in spite of corrective attempts by the manufacturer. Worldwide, approximately 82,000 valves have been implanted and an estimated number of 650 fractures have been reported. A US Congress Committee and investigators established shortcomings on the part of the Food and Drug Administration, and fraud with manufacturing records ('the phantom welder'), inadequately trained personnel, misrepresentation of risks of fracture by the management and reworking of valves rejected in the process of quality control (Committee on Energy and Commerce, 1990; van der Graaf *et al.*, 1998). The manufacturer failed to report fractures to the FDA, while marketing activities were continued despite the awareness of the problems. When it came to communicating the risk of fracture to prescribers and patients, no adequate implant register existed. Therefore, many patients either did not know they carried a BScc valve or could not be tracked for risk information. Although basically an engineering issue, the problem was compounded by inappropriate responses by doctors, hospitals and health authorities (de Mol *et al.*, 1997a). In The Netherlands, heart valve failures were also observed with Hemex Duromedics (Baxter Inc.) and Medtronic Parallel (Medtronic Inc.) valves. Disputes about resources and scientific research requirements inhibited the development of an effective worldwide risk strategy.

A systemic safety management approach needs a structural and political basis in society at large (Cromheecke *et al.*, 1998). Professions are inclined to focus exclusively on the subsystems and tasks they can control and tend to exclusively promote their view as the single risk control solution. In The Netherlands, we were able to overcome public outrage and potential conflicts of interest through the establishment of the so-called Björk-Shiley convexo-concave study group, in which all implanting centres were involved. A register of all patients was established and continuous follow-up, in the sense of a longitudinal cohort study, was carried out (de Mol *et al.*, 1994; van der Graaf *et al.*, 1992). Parallel technical analysis of retrieved valves was carried out by the Delft University of Technology and Rice University, Texas. The clinical records, incident data, and the technical information provided the input for reports by the inter-university working group on cardiovascular implant retrieval analysis. In this working group, pathologists, metallurgists, cardiologists, and surgeons reviewed explanted and fractured valves (de Mol *et al.*, 1997b). Ultimately this work led to the concept of the product life cycle-based safety management and Barrier Analysis, which were developed, between 1992-1997.

In this chapter, first we focus on product life cycle-based safety management for implant failure on the basis of our experience with the BScc valve problem. Second, adverse events and accidents are reviewed and the analyses used to develop a safety management system. Third, the components of the subsystem that represent barriers to undesired scenarios and outcome are reviewed.

TESTING MEDICAL DEVICES

Since June 1998, all medical devices to be used in Europe are supposed to be certified for their safety and efficacy by a notifying body. Industry, health authorities and users have drawn up standards of performance for different classes of device. Clinical tests are required but, especially in the surgical arena, randomised clinically controlled trials are rarely carried out, while the many observational studies provide conflicting information (Horton, 1996). Therefore, safety is only really assessed in long-term observational studies after the devices are in use with patients.

Standards, however, are lagging behind the newest developments and tested devices in real use may not to live up to expectations. As regards in-vivo durability and long-term biocompatiblity, there is little consensus on the test results of implants such as heart valves (de Mol, 1996a). Therefore, the explantation (removal) of implants and subsequent analysis is important to assess whether the degradation process predicted prior to implantation is similar to the observed wear. In the overwhelming majority of cases there is no reason for the explantation and further examination of hip prostheses, pacemakers, breast implants or heart valves. Therefore, only in cases of evident failure of an implant are studies carried out to assess and explain the failure mode. Devices to support patient self-management are even more complex to assess. Apart from the reliability of the device, effective and safe patient-management is also determined by the user who acts interactively with the device. The patient's capability depends on their physical status, training and education, support and confidence in the physician, the device and himself.

Conclusions from these studies will only be valid where several analyses of implants of the same type are carried out and where there are guidelines regarding preservation and analysis of the implant. These data only become meaningful in conjunction with epidemiological data, manufacturing records and comparisons of performance with other brand types. The findings of such studies may have serious financial implications for manufacturers and pose a liability problem for manufacturer and prescriber alike (de Mol and Fielder, 1997a).

A structured approach to investigation of device failures and the control of risk for the remaining implant bearers is therefore required. The observations and conclusions of the failure analysis provide the input for risk control and safety management measures. This interdependence explains why poor failure analysis results in poor damage limitation (de Mol and Fielder, 1997a). The threat of litigation and the fact that the failure analysis may be biased by hindsight generate disputes between interested parties about the observations and analyses. Judicial tests regarding engineering and managerial decisions are especially difficult. Should engineers and manufacturer have known, ten years ago, according to the scientific evidence available at that time, that their provisions to warrant durability were faulty and defective and, if so, to what extent?

From the point of view of safety management, learning, improving and preventing damage are the primary objectives of a failure analysis. Second, safety management has to be executed within a systems approach (Bignell and Fortune, 1984), aiming ultimately at a better design for the system. As the systems approach in healthcare safety is relatively undeveloped, attempts to explain accidents often result in blaming some person or party. This contribution aims to illustrate the value of a systems approach to enhancement of device safety. A transparent and structured approach to analysing device failure is presented which is used in the development of both safety management systems and risk communication strategies.

TREATMENT OF HEART VALVE DISEASE AND VALVE FAILURE

The heart consists of two pump chambers which have an inlet and outlet valve. One chamber sends the supply of oxygenated blood to the various organs such as brain, kidneys, legs etc. The other chamber pumps oxygen-depleted blood from the heart to the lungs, where it is re-oxygenated. The first system is more vulnerable to infections and rheumatic fever, and degenerates faster due to ageing. Generally, younger people have to undergo valve replacement because of valve deformation and leakage due to infection or birth defects, while older people tend to undergo valve replacement for degenerative disease. Progress in technology enables us to carry out open-heart surgery with the aid of a heart-lung machine, in sicker and older people. Valves of biological material such as bovine and porcine pericardium, and even human allografts, are available. However, their limited durability and scarcity mean that the large-scale use of mechanical heart valves is necessary. Mechanical heart valves are designed to outlive the patient in terms of durability. In contrast to biological substitutes, the mechanical heart valves require lifelong anti-coagulation therapy. The level of anticoagulation has to be regularly checked, usually by visiting a special anticoagulant clinic.

Self-management by a finger-prick, however, provides more frequent testing and reduces time-consuming visits to a clinic.

VALVE FAILURE IN A SYSTEM'S PERSPECTIVE

Between April 1993 and April 1997, the Interuniversity Working Group on Cardiovascular Implant Retrieval examined three types of valve failure:

Type 1 failure related to leakage of the valve due to compression, which was later explained as a combination of design shortcoming, surgical error, and special disease. This series of four cases appeared to be an institutional problem.

Type 2 failure was related to the fact that a suture wedged between the ring and the closure disk, which caused impingement or blockage. This failure mode is predominantly a surgical error. The valve cannot open and the patient dies. Since 1982, this event has been reported for that type of valve at a rate of 0.5 % of implantations. In 1997, we studied two cases.

Type 3 failure were the fractured BScc valves, resulting in escape of the disk within the valve, leading to the patient's death. The failure mode is considered a technical shortcoming, and is the type of failure discussed in this chapter. Due to the number of failures of the BScc valve (type 3) and the duration of the problem (since 1979), we were able to identify the steps in the failure cascade.

BARRIER ANALYSIS OF THE BSCC FAILURE

The descriptions that follow of the shortcomings in the system mark barriers which were supposed to prevent the failure in the first place, or at least to reduce the damage toll to patients and the system. Barrier analysis may be used to investigate accidents, considering the reasons for the failure of barriers and whether sufficient barriers exist. Although the concept was developed to investigate the impact of physical violence or energy on vulnerable objects (e.g. people), barriers may be also administrative. Another potential of barrier analysis lies in its focus on human error to be overcome by reinforcing barriers or designing more reliable barriers to decrease vulnerability. Referring to the description of the string of failures and the product life cycle based system, the connections between components are similar to barriers.

a) The primary cause of BScc valve failure was fatigue due to design and manufacturing flaws. Originally, the valve had two struts, which were welded into the flange. Due to a relatively low but serious number of strut fractures, it was decided to make the major strut out of one piece and to weld the minor strut. Although never confirmed by clinical tests, the manufacturer also decided to enlarge the opening angle and to change the flat disk into a convexo-concave-shaped disk. Although welding of the alloy used in this ring was, even then, a substandard technique, the new design requirements asked for a special welding procedure, which made the welding even more critical. Therefore, welding could not even at that time be considered an appropriate technology (van der Graaf *et al.*, 1992; de Mol *et al.*, 1997b).

b) Lack of training and qualified personnel to carry out the welding resulted in numerous valves of poor quality and a high rate of rejection. Drug and alcohol abuse was also discovered among factory workers during manufacturing, which was a continuous, 24-hour operation.

c) The valve was a commercial success thanks to aggressive marketing. Reports of strut fracture were known to the manufacturer, but valves that were not accepted by quality control were repolished or remilled and declared acceptable for implantation.

d) In spite of FDA (Food and Drug Administration) orders, the manufacturer refused to adjust the quality control procedures.

e) Due to shortcomings within the FDA, no adequate measures were instituted and the management was able to deliberately mislead the healthcare authorities.

f) Due to the lack of procedures on authority and communications between the FDA and the Dutch health inspectorate, valves that were prohibited for the USA market could still be implanted in The Netherlands.

g) Cardiac surgeons allowed themselves to be impressed by the tough marketing approach of the manufacturer. Claims of superiority were never proven but made this valve commercially one of the most successful.

h) The risk control of this problem was initially left completely to the manufacturer in the hope that they were monitoring any problems worldwide. Although cardiac surgeons are also supposed to be in charge of risk control, they delegated this responsibility to cardiologists, who in turn had their own responsibilities.

i) There was no register of implanted valves or patients, either in the hospital or with the manufacturer. No follow-up was carried out. In The Netherlands, approximately 2,300 valves were implanted and it took 16 fractures and 14 deaths before the problem in our small country became clear.

j) The problem was played down by health authorities, manufacturer, and the cardiac profession. Hard data on the number of cases and the etiology of failure remained scarce or were deliberately made confusing. The manufacturer approached cardiac surgeons and health authorities with reassuring, and misleading '*Dear Doctor*' letters.

k) Risk communication was extremely diffuse and provided only on an occasional basis by all parties involved, including consumer organisations. All media, from consultation room to prime-time television, were used. So far, only the responsibility of the manufacturer and his parent Pfizer Inc. has been established. Criminal prosecution for that could be settled with 20 million U.S. dollars.

l) Patients with BScc implants arrived at a class action settlement with Pfizer Inc. on behalf of Shiley Inc. In the case of a strut fracture, BScc carriers were entitled to a fixed amount of compensation, which differed between countries and carriers. The settlement also provided 17 million dollars for research in order to develop diagnostic tools in order to monitor the technical status of the valve. So far, in spite of spending 37 million dollars in a five-year period, no useful or beneficial medical strategy for patients has been developed.

m) The settlement between carriers and manufacturer is supposed to be supervised by a U.S. judge. The stakes for the lawyers representing the class and Pfizer are high. Regarding the technical and 'scientific' implementation, a supervisory panel of scientists appointed by the parties is taking care of so-called clinical guidelines and future scientific research. The local professional communities, who usually draw up practice guidelines, remain excluded.

In 1995 and 1997, the seven patients who suffered a BScc strut fracture died, in spite of the two risk control strategies (de Mol and Fielder, 1997a).

THE PRODUCT LIFE CYCLE-BASED SAFETY MANAGEMENT SYSTEM

The industrial concept of risk and quality management can also be applied to device and implantation manufacturing (Bignell and Fortune, 1984; Perrow, 1987; Wagenaar and van de Schrier, 1997). The product life cycle-based safety management system includes all persons, hospital departments, and healthcare authorities involved with a product. This system is divided into four subsystems, which correspond with phases according to the product's life cycle.

Phase A: Design and manufacturing

In this phase, direct involvement with design and manufacturing is provided by designers, employers, and the quality assurance division. However, interests related to the design and manufacturing process are also attributed to the parent company, venture capitalist funding, subcontractors, unions, and share holders.

Phase B: Regulation and marketing

Although a marketing strategy is developed as soon as a product is taking shape, access to the market is determined by the regulatory authorities. In this phase, user instructions and proper indications for use are developed and tested. The secondary interests to the process lie with the licensing agency, marketing organisation, distributing organisation and clinical research institutes.

Phase C: Implantation and control of patient risks

In this phase, implantation of the device takes place. In the case of heart valves, the implantation centre is also the referral centre where problems after implantation must be diagnosed and resolved. The implementation of the indication for implantation, user instructions, information to patients, and provisions for follow-up take place in this phase.

In phase C, product handling is carried out by the purchasing department, operating room storage, all operating room (OR) personnel, surgeons, and in a remote sense, by the team providing the aftercare. The secondary interests relating to the process lie with hospital organisation and management, budget control section, insurance company, participating specialities such as cardiology and physiotherapy, and the inpatients complaint agency.

Phase D: Performance and follow-up

The device is now carried by the patient and serves its purpose. However, adjustments and maintenance are carried out within or without a planned follow-up scheme. Only active devices, such as pacemakers, can be adjusted. However, we know that devices can migrate or show minor changes, which can be diagnosed on X-ray, as is the case with hip prostheses and breast implants. In this phase, an assessment has to be made as to whether the implants are fulfilling their expectations, from the point of view of the carrier as well as the healthcare provider. Registration, follow-up, and early-warning and quick-rating schemes have to be made operational in this phase.

Figure 10.1 gives a more detailed overview of the processes controlled by persons and institutions. The authorities involved are subdivided into pro subsystem or life cycle phase, and connected to each other as components. The primary involvement with the product lies with the patients, the family doctor, or the controlling specialists in the community hospitals. The secondary interests lie with the health authorities, which, together with manufacturer and implanting hospital, are supposed to carry out the postmarketing surveillance. Pathologists, ambulance services, and patient/consumer organisations may also have an interest when problems arise in this phase. Action by these secondary interested parties is essential for acceptable and successful intervention in case of failure of the device. They are important as they represent the potential sources of conflict of interest. The way these people and organisations interact on the basis of their task to control risk provide the foundation for application of the barrier concept (Kirwan and Ainsworth, 1993).

	PRODUCT LIFE CYCLE-BASED SAFETY MANAGEMENT HAZARD BARRIER ANALYSIS			
	A **Design /** **Manufacturing**	**B** **Certification /** **Marketing**	**C** **Implantation**	**D** **Follow-up**
Handling				
Risk Assessment Risk Control Engineering Evaluation	Science Design Engineering Production	Technical Tests Clinical Tests Agency Distribution	Purchase Referral Informed Consent Surgery Postoperative Care	Patient Family Doctor Surgeon Ambulance ER / Hospitals Retrieval Analysis
Interests				
Financial Legal	Managers Financiers Scientists	Authorities + A	Patients Doctors Care Insurers + A & B	Patients & Relatives Damage Insurers Experts Lawyers Media + A & B & C

Figure 10.1 The product life cycle-based safety management system. It includes all persons, hospital departments, and healthcare authorities involved with a product.

Designing barriers for protection is difficult and complex, requiring input from designers (phase A), safety people (phase B), and operators (Phase C), and have to be tested in the accident-prone environment (Phase D). The accident analysis approach based on barrier analysis also provides a strong basis for the product life cycle-based safety management system.

ACCIDENT REPORTS, ANALYSIS AND RISK PERCEPTION

A product life-cycle safety management system approach is a generic framework which describes, understands and anticipates people, interests and authorities in the area of safety maintenance and risk control. It may be applied to classes of events related to devices or to equipment, which may have a shorter or longer life cycle.

Prior to applying the product life cycle-based concept, a phase of recognition has to be passed. The events must have been primarily attributed to device failure, substantial number events must have occurred and there must have been a substantial threat to patients. Large-scale failure of devices may have a large or small time window. When the adverse events are scattered around the world in several centres, the number of failures and the effectiveness of a risk control strategy are difficult to assess. Public outrage may mobilize consumer organisations but may also cause large conflicts of interest, hampering solutions. However, when a product life cycle-based safety management system as a concept is adopted, one may anticipate frictions as summarised above.

Therefore, incident reporting and analysis remain the central means of both discovering and learning from adverse events. Within the framework of postmarketing surveillance and duty to follow up, adequate incident reporting at higher aggregation level provides the data essential for activating supra-institutional risk control by means of product life-cycle based safety management. Our group developed a systematic incident identification system, an easy-to-handle digital form, which provides data for analysis and the maintenance of a register (Wagenaar and van de Schrier, 1997).

Temporary paralysis due to thromboembolic events is a common complication or performance endpoint in mechanical heart valve failure. The rate of thromboembolism is considered a measure of technical performance. However, we found that in several cases, in which at first sight the mere presence of a valve was held responsible for the complication, shortcomings in patient management were partly responsible for the adverse outcome. Of course, the presence of a mechanical heart valve remains under all circumstances a dominant risk factor, which narrows the safety margins.

The type of failure determines the type of action to be taken by doctors and patients. The wedging of a suture was considered by surgeons as an 'all-in-the-game' event, which was considered completely unacceptable by the patient. This results in a continuation of the usual practise by surgeons, but patients will sue the hospital and/or the manufacturer for negligence and so far they have done that successfully (Vincent *et al.*, 1994).

In conclusion, accident monitoring and risk perception determine largely whether the product life-cycle systems approach will be activated. However, once operationalised, actions and effects do occur within subsystems and components. This process follows basically the Risk Assessment and Control cycle as described by Hale (1995). In the BScc application nearly all relevant parties eventually embarked on effective actions. However, the timing, communication and effectiveness of the actions remained questionable. Risk communication and effective assessment of control actions therefore need further description.

THE CONTROL STRATEGIES AND RISK COMMUNICATION

Risk control for medical implants is extremely complicated. In case of failures and threats to the interests of stakeholders within the subsystems of the product life cycle, logical alliances and agreements may fail completely when other subsystems and components are not taken into consideration. Good examples are the '*Dear Doctor*' letters of the manufacturer in order to minimise the risk and to protect the interest of shareholders (Fielder, 1993, 1994). The manufacturer's information to health authorities, doctors and patients was established to be misleading, due to the conflict of interest between all parties involved. But positive actions may also be frustrated by one-direction communication. Parts of the settlement agreement between patients and manufacturer regarding new research and indications for operative treatment were never implemented, because the health authorities and medical profession were not included. With respect to scientific approaches of risk estimation, the medical profession will accept these new findings only if they are scientifically credible and when all prerequisites for transforming these findings into new practise guidelines have been fulfilled. The health authorities on the other hand, are left with a public-health problem in the sense that they have to care for the patients falling victim to outlet strut fractures and the costs of dealing with the ongoing problem.

As society and life are full of risks, risk communication mainly serves the purpose of increasing the acceptance of risk with the parties involved (Bignell and Fortune, 1984; Perrow, 1987; Calman, 1996; Fitzpatrick, 1996). In the case of the BScc valve carriers, the risk of outlet strut fracture has been established by 'body counting'. The population at risk was known, as was the number of documented outlet strut fracture. The risk of fracture depended on the opening angle, the age of the patient, the size of the valve, and the position of the valve in the heart. The risk varied from 0.5% to 2% per year (van der Graaf *et al.*, 1992). Technical research revealed that there was a tremendous variation in fracture patterns (de Mol *et al.*, 1997b). It is virtually impossible to make any prediction within relevant time frames of months to one year. Given the size of the substrate it is unlikely that, with conventional diagnostic tools, prefracture signals can be detected. Therefore, basically two risk control strategies were available (Koornneef *et al.*, 1996):

1) Preventive explantation of the valve

In this strategy, the immediate risk of the reoperation to remove the risky heart valve varies from 2 to 5% and has to be balanced against the cumulative risk of fracture within the estimated life expectancy of the patient.

2) The run-for-your-life option

When there is no obvious gain of life expectancy after balancing the risks the patient is left with the 'run-for-your-life' option which requires immediate access to cardiac surgical care in the event of failure. However, this strategy depends on an early diagnosis by lay people in the community, availability of ambulance and helicopter services, immediate referral to a cardiac surgical centre and instant emergency reoperation. Past experience with the series of seven consecutive deaths makes clear that ambulance services, community hospitals, family practitioner, and cardiac surgical centre do not co-operate and communicate adequately. In all cases, the patient himself or the relatives were able to make the instant diagnosis of strut fracture and valve failure, but they were simply ignored by the experts.

When taking a closer look at the parties involved in emergency care in The Netherlands, and the way tasks and obligations are bureaucratically separated and fragmented, it becomes obvious that survival depends largely on luck and the personal strength of the patient. Ambulance drivers are daily briefed on where to bring cardiac emergency cases and may refuse to transport patients dying from a valve fracture to a cardiac surgical unit. Seven deaths in a row obviously diminish the credibility of the medical authorities in the handling of the crisis (de Mol and Fielder, 1997a; Koornneef *et al.*, 1996; Sandman, 1991).

The patient's quality of life may be affected by carrying a risky device continuously and receiving disquieting messages from the media (Fielder, 1994; Kallewaard *et al.*, 1997). Risk communication may improve communication and effectiveness of risk control strategies and increase the acceptance of the residual risks to the patient (risk taker), the doctor (risk controller) and the public (justice). A risk communication programme should serve the following objectives:

i)   awareness of the danger;

(ii)   information with respect to the individual exposure;

(iii)   counselling with respect to risk control and prevention;
(iv)   providing new information in order to decrease uncertainty;
(v)   ensuring that solutions accord with principles of justice.

The societal impact of dangers and the willingness to embark on a risk communication and control strategy depend on the safety culture.   As medical devices are designed and manufactured with the aim of zero failure and high durability, the safety culture with respect to the technical performance is highly developed in phase A and phase B. However, in phase C and phase D, the primary controllers of risk and performance of the device have to monitor many other implants. They therefore rely heavily on the intrinsic safety generated in phases A and B, though the awareness and expression of safety culture in phases C and D differ in terms of intensity and effectiveness.

The product life cycle-based safety management system provides a model that may guide the contents of the message as well as the number of people / components to be informed in order to achieve the effect of re-enforcing barriers, changing duties in order to co-operate effectively and communicating the nature of the risk. So, sender, receiver, copyholders, and contents of the message may be guided by the product life cycle-based safety management system. The system also allows predictions on acceptance of the message as risk perception and safety culture / awareness of the parties can be described.

SYSTEMS CONTROL AND ASSESSMENT

Systems Control

Safety management is expensive and demands many resources, especially during a crisis. Effective decision making relies on adequate information being available. Safety crises in relation to implants were characterised by incomplete data and uncertainty regarding risks and the effectiveness of risk control strategies. Therefore, within the subsystems or product life cycle phases, platforms must be created with a hierarchy of risk control. We propose that in phase A the management of a manufacturing company is in charge, in phase B the health authority, in phase C the implanting physician, and in phase D the controlling physician closest to the patient.

Reviewing the problems with the BScc valves, the root causes of failure in the various subsystems varied. In phase A, the management was fraudulent, in phase B, the health authorities were incompetent, in phase C, the physicians in charge were ignorant, and in phase D, the general practitioner or controlling cardiologist was still uninformed and unaware. In phase D, such a dedicated relationship is lacking as attending physicians take care of many risks, which fortunately rarely materialise and therefore cannot take on the task of monitoring specific devices, though they should report failures. In terms of system control, an information and communication platform is required as well as knowledge of devices, risks, and tools to estimate risks and their consequences. In phase C, specialities, such as cardiovascular surgery, plastic surgery, and orthopaedic surgery, may create their own statutory safety committees based on selfregulation. These rulings relate to topics such as a register of patients, follow-up criteria to carry out clinical studies with devices, and guidelines on dealing with technical and marketing information provided by manufacturers.

In phase B, health authorities may, as with the licensing process for drugs, draw up regulatory and technical committees to assess devices. In phase A, the risk of product liability and competition on safety and performance are supposed to force the manufacturer to comply with the safety standards. A safety board for medical devices should have the expertise to deal with the actual risk control within the system but also to execute the political and societal demands from the point of view of individual and public healthcare.

Assessment of Effectiveness

The efficacy of the model can only be finally assessed by its outcome. For this purpose, and applied to the BScc valve problem, Koornneef *et al.* describe a risk intensity assessment model (RIA). Such a model enables the assessment of the level of system integrity as a threshold for containing damage due to device failure. The model uses the parameters of the former DIN 19250 standard:

1. The 'consequence/risk' parameter, reflecting the seriousness of harm of loss, which varies from minor injury to a catastrophe with many fatalities.
2. The 'frequency and exposure-time risk' parameter, reflecting duration of exposure to harmful conditions, which may vary from seldom to permanent.
3. The 'possibility of avoiding risk' parameter, reflecting options to divert/control imminent danger, which varies from possible under certain conditions to hardly possible.
4. The 'probability of risk realisation' parameter, reflecting prevalence of failure, which may vary from a very low probability to a relatively high probability.

Risk control measurements may be directed towards one or several of these thresholds, which should result in reinforcement of the system integrity and an overall reduction of potential injury and damage.

The RIA model indicated that the preventive replacement strategy of risky BScc valves was the strategy to be preferred, but Dutch cardiac surgical centres took a different approach. Some centres opted for many preventive reoperations of the valve, others gave preference to explantation of the valves most at risk and the wait-and-see options for others. The latter group paid a higher death toll in outlet strut fracture (six of the seven deaths, the other death refused to be operated on even though it was recommended) and is now forced to carry out more reoperations, at still higher risk, as patients have grown older. So, three years later it is confirmed that according to the point of view of systems control, preventive explantation has provided the most effective damage control.

We must be aware that the medical speciality primarily focus on strategies aimed at individuals. Risk strategies for populations belong to the public health sector, which did not recognise the BScc problem. However, on an individual basis, it is the decision of the doctor and the patient to opt for one of the two strategies, based on the best information available. This assumes that the best information is available to the decision-making doctor and patient, information with which they feel confident, as it is generated within their own professional discipline, though it may not always be the best available (de Mol and Fielder, 1997a; Fielder, 1994 and 1996).

RESOURCES AND MULTIDISCIPLINARY RESEARCH: THE NEED FOR A NATIONAL DEVICE SAFETY BOARD

Reporting, analysing and learning from adverse event reports is expensive, especially with large-scale enterprises. Usually, funding for prevention is only allocated where it can be attributed to the price of a device. Pre-implant testing is an accepted manufacturing cost. The costs of maintaining a register of heart valve carriers are still not determined or allocated to any party. Are these costs to be paid by the manufacturer, institution, or any other authority? This raises questions about the control, confidentiality, the extent of a register and its cost effectiveness. Research might reveal not only shortcomings on the part of the manufacturer, but also on the part of health authorities and doctors.

Doctors might anticipate questions about why they selected the BScc valve amongst others, why they ignored early reports on strut fracture, why they kept the extent of the problem from patients at risk and how they judged the technical and clinical research supporting the market approval of the BScc valve. These questions usually arise when a design or material failure cause implant dysfunction (de Mol and van Gaalen, 1996b). In the BScc case, it could be argued that the manufacturer should promote and fund technical research to confirm the liability, clarify the extent of the problem, and result in the recognition of many cases to be compensated. On the other hand, critical research carried out by an interested party will lack scientific credibility and objectivity. However, health authorities that are publicly funded were also reluctant to fund investigation. As it is obvious that the manufacturer is liable for the damages, the authorities refused to take any funding initiative. They referred to the legal obligation of the manufacturer, who in his turn had is own damage control agenda.

In The Netherlands a small grant was only made available from the Health Authority after the threat of a legal procedure by the Consumer Organisation. This provided the basis for substantial technical and epidemiological research, providing some basic information to enhance decision making, in spite of its chronic under-funding. For less spectacular device failures, dedicated research programmes to fill the gaps of knowledge are still lacking. Lack of funding and delays in obtaining information are hampering the development of risk control strategies.

Procedures to recognise and analyse serial device and implant failures will be well founded when based on the product life cycle-based management system. Involvement of public bodies to facilitate research, funding and execution of strategies can be achieved only if a succinct and objective presentation is made by the parties involved. This requires a proactive and continuous effort to assure the safety of implants and devices. To avoid difficulties with access and bureaucracy, national agencies or safety boards, similar to the Transportation Safety Boards or Pharma Vigilance System, should be instituted.

CONCLUSIONS

We demonstrated with the BScc valve failures the value of the concept of product life cycle-based safety management at the supra-institutional level. Incident reporting, incident analysis and risk perception largely determine the threshold for institutional or supra-institutional safety management. Safety management identifies the key players, a hierarchy of risk control, and guides the content and flow of risk communication. Last, but not least, it discriminates between parties really 'touching' the implant and parties taking a recognised societal interest in the implantation process. The potential for conflicts of interests can be clarified and anticipated. In close conjunction, the risk intensity assessment model enables estimations about the effectiveness of damage control. For a device such as CoaguChek®, which also enables patient self-management of anticoagulant therapy, extra classes of risks, conflict of interests and pitfalls in communication can be identified.

Putting these concepts into practice depends largely on public awareness, political responsibility and legal liability. Lack of knowledge, funding and safety management tools can be overcome, once a proactive approach is chosen by the key role players in the life cycle phases: the manufacturer (A), the Health Authority (B), the Doctor (C) and the patient (D). A national device safety board could provide the administrative platform to harbour knowledge, experience and factual guidance of safety management.

REFERENCES

Bignell, V., and J. Fortune (1984). *Understanding system failures*. Manchester University Press, Manchester.

Black, J. (1996). Implant retrieval: an overview of goals and perspectives. *Int. J. Risk & Safety in Med.,* 99-105.

Committee on Energy and Commerce. U.S. House of Representatives. (1990). *The Björk-Shiley heart valve: "Earn as You Learn". Shiley Inc.'s breach of the honour system and FDA's failure in medical device regulation.* U.S.GPO 26-766, Feb. Washington.

Calman, K. C. (1996). Cancer: science and society and the communication of risk. *B.M.J.,* **313,** 799-802.

Cromheecke, M. E., P. J. Overkamp, B. A. de Mol, G. L. van Gaalen, A. E. Becker (1998). Retrieval analysis of mechanical heart valves: Impact on design and clinical practice. *Artif. Organs,* **22**(9), 794-799.

de Mol, B. A., M. Kallewaard, R. B. McLellen, L. A. van Herwerden, J. J. Defauw, and Y. van der Graaf (1994). Single-leg fractures in explanted Björk-Shiley valves. *Lancet,* **343,** 9-12.

de Mol, B. A., F. Koornneef and G. L. van Gaalen (1995). What can be done to improve the safety of heart valves? *Int. J. Risk & Safety in Med.,* **6,** 157-168.

de Mol, B. A. (1996a). Retrieval analysis of cardiovascular implants. *Int. J. Risk and Safety Med.,* **8,** 119-123.

de Mol, B. A. and G. L. van Gaalen (1996b). The editor's corner: Biomaterials Crisis in the Medical Device Industry: Is litigation the only cause? *J Biomed Mater Res.,* **33,** 53-54.

de Mol, B. A. and J. H. Fielder (1997a). Systemic accident analysis of deaths due to failed Bjork-Shiley heart valves. *Int. J. Risk and Safety Med.,* **10,** 243-247.

de Mol, B. A., P. J. Overkamp, G. L. van Gaalen and A. E. Becker (1997b). Non-destructive assessment of 62 Dutch Björk-Shiley convexo-concave heart valves. *Eur. J. Cardio-thorac. Surgery,* **11,** 703-709.

Fielder, J. H. (1993). Getting the bad news about your artificial heart valve. *Hastings Center Report,* **23**(2), 22-28.

Fielder, J. H. (1994). More bad news about Björk-Shiley c/c heart valves. *IEEE Engin. & Med. Biol.,* 182-4.

Fitzpatrick, R. (1996). Telling patients there is nothing wrong. *B.M.J.*, **313**, 311-312.

Hale, A. R. (1995). In: *Management of safety, health and environment: Risk assessment and control*, 21-211. MoSHE Manual, Top Tech Studies. Delft

Hasenkam, J. M., H. H. Kimose, L. Knudsen, H. Grønnesby, J. Halborg, T. D. Christensen, J. Attermann and H. K. Filegaard (1997). Self management of oral anticoagulant therapy after heart valve replacement. *Eur. J. Cardio-thorac Surgery*, **11**(5), 935-942.

Horton, R. (1996). Surgical Research a comic opera: questions, but few answers. *Lancet*, **347**, 984-985.

Kallewaard, M., J. J. Defauw, and Y. van der Graaf (1997). Psychological distress among Björk-Shiley cc valve recipients: the impact of information. *Heart*

Kirwan, B. and L. K. Ainsworth (1993). *A guide to task analysis*. 169-178. Taylor and Francis, London.

Koornneef, F., G. L. van Gaalen and B. A. de Mol (1996). A risk assessment and control model for the failing Björk-Shiley convexo-concave heart valve. *Int. J. Tech. Assess. in Health Care*, **12**, 141-145.

Koornneef, F. and A. R. Hale (1997). Learning from incidents at work. In: *Human factors in safety critical systems*. (F. Redmill, J. Rajan, eds.). Butterworth Heinemann, Oxford.

Laffel, G. and D. Blumenthal (1989). The case for using industrial quality management science in health care organizations. *J.A.M.A.*, **262**, 2869-2873.

Perrow, Ch. (1987). *Normal accidents. Living with high-risk technologies*. Basic Book Publ. Inc., New York.

Sandman, P. M. (1991). Emerging communication responsibilities of epidemiologists. *J. Clin. Epid.*, **44** (suppl. 1), 41S-45S.

Starr, A. (1986). The Thoracic Surgical Industrial Complex. *Ann. Thorac. Surgery*, **42**,124-132.

van der Graaf, Y., F. de Waard, L. A. van Herwerden, and J. J. Defauw (1992). Risk of strut fracture of Björk-Shiley valves. *Lancet*, **339**, 257-261.

van der Graaf, Y., M. Kallewaard and A. Algra (1998). Chronicle of a faulty heart valve prosthesis. *Ned. Tijdschr. Geneeskd.*, **142**, 1645-1648.

Vincent, C. A., M. Young and A. Philips (1994). Why do people sue doctors? A study of patients and relatives taking legal action. *Lancet*, **343**, 1609-1613.

Wagenaar, W. A. and J. van de Schrier (1997). Accident analysis: the goal and how to get there. *Safety Science*, **26**, 25-33.

CHAPTER 11

EARLY EVALUATION OF NEW TECHNOLOGIES: THE CASE FOR MOBILE MULTIMEDIA COMMUNICATIONS IN EMERGENCY MEDICINE.

Fred W.G. van den Anker, Delft University of Technology, The Netherlands
Rob A. Lichtveld, Utrecht Ambulance Service, The Netherlands

EARLY EVALUATION OF NEW TECHNOLOGIES

Introduction

On October 27th 1992 the computerised command-and-control system operated by the London Ambulance Service (LAS) broke down. As a result of this failure, patients had to wait many hours for an ambulance. The outcomes of the LAS project involving the computerisation of control-room operations are radically different from the successful introduction of a similar computer despatch system at the Greater Manchester Ambulance Service (GMAS). The contrasting outcomes can be attributed to management failures and a technology-driven approach at the London Ambulance Service, as opposed to a user-involved design approach with strong commitment from the management in Manchester (Wastell and Cooper, 1996).

What is apparent from the Inquiry Team's investigation of the London Ambulance Service disaster is that neither the Computer Aided Despatch (CAD) system itself, nor its users, were ready for full implementation on 26 October 1992 (Finkelstein, 1995). The system was incomplete and not fully tested. Unrealistic timetables were set out without consultation and commitment of those involved. There was incomplete ownership of the system by the users, who had no confidence in the system and were not fully trained. The initiatives undertaken by management before implementation worsened what was already a cultural climate of mistrust and poor communications. Moreover, the CAD system did not fit the organisational structure and operational procedures. Satisfactory implementation of the system required changes to a number of existing working practices. However, senior management believed that implementation of the system would, in itself, bring about these changes.

This example shows several points related to this contribution: (1) the need to consider human, social as well as organisational factors when introducing new technologies; (2) to involve the users themselves in the development process, and (3) the importance of looking in advance for problems that may arise by putting new technologies to work, instead of just waiting for them to happen.

However, the design-oriented, prospective assessment of positive and negative consequences of new technologies for work and organisation still lacks a sound methodology. This is especially true for the evaluation of the potential problems and risks introduced by future technologies such as mobile multimedia communications, which will be discussed in this contribution. Mobile multimedia communications enable a mobile worker to communicate with another worker, not only through audio/ speech and data, but through video as well. Due to bandwidth limitations, the technology for mobile multimedia communications is not yet available, and for that reason it is not yet clear which kind of applications could be useful, where and for whom, and which problems and risks they may bring about. Technology assessment in this stage of development offers a means to prevent future risks and unsuccessful implementations, but there is great uncertainty involved in evaluating a future situation.

To support the design process from the beginning, a method is necessary to identify, represent and evaluate potentially useful applications and their influence on work activities. More specifically, the major gap lies in the availability of a way to create representations of future 'socio-technical' systems which the potential users and other stakeholders can use to explore individual, social and organizational implications (Eason *et al.*, 1996). In a case study on the usefulness of mobile multimedia communications for emergency medicine, we have tried to fill this gap by developing scenarios offering the potential user community a concrete vision of their future work activities. Participatory, worker-involved evaluation of these envisioned work activities should set the stage for safe and effective systems design in an early phase of the development cycle.

Early, Scenario-based Evaluation

The earlier in the design process a system is evaluated, the more flexibility there will be with respect to changes in design. The evaluation of an already implemented system does not leave much space for major changes. There is a need for quick and cost efficient methods to support the exploration of socio-technical alternatives and requirements before the actual design of a system. Most current user-centered methods show major deficiencies with respect to such an early, contextual assessment of design concepts.

Traditional methods for gathering system requirements that are based on a waterfall model of systems development (Figure 11.1) do not incorporate extensive evaluation of design concepts in an early stage. They tend to rely on the possibility of a precise and direct specification of system requirements on the basis of an analysis of the application domain. However, a direct translation of user needs to formalised system requirements is problematic, since needs and requirements often only become apparent when the system is used. Thus, current user-centered methods often use some form of prototype to let users interact with the new system in an early stage of development. However, these more iterative approaches that use early prototyping and evaluation methods like usability testing are at that stage already rather focused on the refinement of user interfaces. With their emphasis on individual human-computer interaction, they do not leave much space for analyzing technological and organisational alternatives. The tendency within the human factors and ergonomics community is to look for usability, i.e. the system's ease of use for individual users and tasks, and to overlook the system's usefulness for the collective organisation of work activities. However, the successful introduction of telematics systems, communication technologies and systems for computer-supported co-operative work is much more dependent on the ability to take into account social and organisational factors than do stand-alone computer systems.

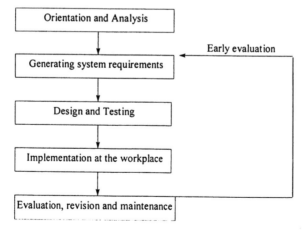

Figure 11.1 In the waterfall model of systems development each phase is completed before the next one starts. Positioning evaluation early in the development cycle allows us to generate requirements on the basis of an assessment of expected implementation problems of preliminary design concepts.

The social and organisational context of work should not only be taken into account in the analysis of the application domain, but also in the generation of system requirements and in the actual design process. The existing work situation will often change or be required to change by the introduction of new technologies. Besides that, the work situation may have changed by the time the technology becomes available and the applications are developed. Therefore, the system requirements should not only concern the technology, but also the work context itself, i.e. the user roles and tasks, the division of labour, communication and co-ordination patterns and the organisational context (e.g. communication and action procedures, division of responsibilities). In fact, future systems design should be based on an analysis and evaluation of the expected and desired future, and not on the existing work situation.

In-depth analysis of the current situation might be of limited value when a new system is expected to introduce considerable change. In the case of future technologies such as mobile multimedia communications, there is great uncertainty with respect to the future work activities that the new technology enables, i.e. useful applications, the users and the tasks to be supported have yet to be defined. Involving users in the design process, as in the Scandinavian participatory design approach (see, for instance, Greenbaum and Kyng, 1991; Schuler and Namioka, 1993), can be especially useful when there are many unknowns about the use of a new technology and its impact on work activities. Besides the objective of democratisation of work and user satisfaction, the (potential) users with different interests in the system can be a valuable source of knowledge with respect to the possibilities and impossibilities of new work activities.

However, the problem is how this knowledge about their future needs and requirements can be generated accurately when potential users and other stakeholders have never used or even imagined the new technological possibilities. To face this problem we have developed an approach that consists of several steps involving the generation and evaluation of a future scenario. The scenario offers the potential user community a concrete vision of their future work activities, not as a prediction of the most likely future, but as a means to think about and discuss future work and the usefulness of new technologies.

No technology is useful in itself. Its usefulness depends on the kind and area of application, and the characteristics of the specific work context to which it is applied. Thus, before the scenario is written, potentially useful applications are identified and the particular 'context of use' is analysed. The application of the future technology and the current work situation form the basis for the development of the future work scenario. The scenario sketches a new interaction process between the actors, some of whom are using the new technology. The future work scenario is assessed by the workers involved on its expected outcomes, the opportunities and limitations for performing their tasks and the problems and risks involved in realising the future work activities. On the basis of the expected and desired outcomes and changes in work and organisation, a new vision on future work and technology may be generated, leading to a different scenario (in terms of the specific users, tasks to be supported, and the social and physical usage environment).

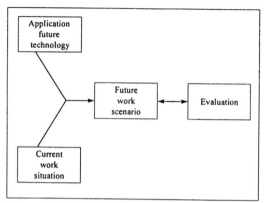

Figure 11.2 The process of early, scenario-based evaluation

Applied to the field of emergency medicine, this approach should lead to a first assessment of the potential contribution of mobile multimedia communications to medical emergency response: its opportunities, the problems and risks it introduces, and the preliminary contextual design requirements as regards safe and effective patient treatment with mobile multimedia communications.

MOBILE MULTIMEDIA COMMUNICATIONS FOR EMERGENCY MEDICINE?

Mobile Multimedia Communications: An Orientation

With the forthcoming European UMTS (Universal Mobile Telecommunications System) standard for mobile communications, which will enable wireless multimedia communications, we should ask ourselves what kind of applications of mobile multimedia communications could be useful for which particular users, tasks and work settings. So far, there has been very little empirical support that rich media such as video-conferencing improve task performance (e.g. Gale, 1990; Rice, 1992). This could be due to the limited functionality that has so far been given to video communications: substituting face-to-face contact by video-conferencing to support the communication process as a goal in itself. However, to conceive of communication as a means to enhance the safe, effective and efficient performance of (physical) tasks is crucial to mobile domains such as emergency medicine. Therefore, we have taken a more task- or action-oriented approach to the identification of useful mobile multimedia applications in terms of the kind of work, tasks and users it could support, and the functionality given to multimedia communications (Van den Anker and Arnold, 1997).

In particular, the 'action regulation theory' (Hacker, 1986; Rasmussen, 1983; Reason, 1990), has been useful in taking a different direction. This theory of human performance and problem solving behaviour makes a distinction between different levels of action regulation. At the skill-based level of performance, familiar tasks are performed in an automatic way. When a problem occurs and the problem is familiar, it can be solved at the rule-based level. However, when the problem situation is new and no routine procedures are available to solve it, the problem solver has to make a conscious analysis of the problem and possible solutions at the knowledge-based level of action regulation. Mobile multimedia communications can play an important role in supporting task performance at the knowledge-based level: those situations in which the mobile worker is faced with complex problems that can not be solved by known procedures (Van den Anker and Arnold, 1998). At this knowledge-based level of task performance, additional expertise from a distance may compensate for the mobile worker's lack of knowledge and skills. This creates a situation of co-operative problem solving.

The usefulness of mobile multimedia communications will depend on the degree to which it facilitates the co-operative problem solving process between the mobile worker and the remote expert. To support the process of collaborative problem solving and task performance, multimedia can be used to show task- or problem-related information, e.g. by means of 'video-as-data' (Nardi *et al.*, 1996). Rather than showing 'talking heads' through video-conferencing, the object of task performance (e.g. the patient) and the actions of the worker towards the object (patient treatment) can be made visible to a remote expert. The shared problem space enables the expert to perceive (see and hear) the local problem, to share knowledge, and to direct and verify the local actions towards a solution. This real-time delivery of remote expertise to mobile settings takes us a step further in the growing area of tele-medicine (e.g. teleconsultation between hospitals, tele-radiology, remote physiological monitoring and home care).

The delivery of remote expertise through mobile multimedia communications can be particularly useful for dealing with critical situations in emergency medicine. Early treatment is crucial in these cases. At present a mobile medical team - a nurse and a physician - is called in for help if the ambulance personnel are unable to handle the situation by themselves. This is for instance the case if hard intubations or surgical coniotomy are necessary. Instead of the time-consuming procedure of going to the place of incident by ambulance or helicopter, the hospital physician can deliver his expertise from a distance, supported by data and video communications, as illustrated in figure 11.3.

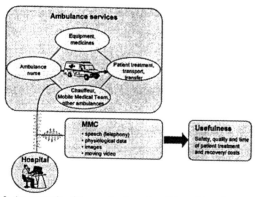

Figure 11.3 An example of the application of mobile multimedia communications

In the current Dutch situation, mobile communications are only used for despatching, co-ordination between the ambulance and the despatch centre, and for the pre-announcement of the patient's vital data, e.g. the traumascore, in order to enable early preparations in the hospital. Mobile communications through multimedia could provide the basis for effective remote support from the hospital to assist the workers on the spot in diagnosing, decision making and/or the physical performance of complex tasks. This may require the hospital physicians and local emergency services to co-ordinate their activities in a synchronous way.

This situation of co-operative problem solving introduces specific problems. Can a diagnosis be made by a remote physician when he has a limited view on the problem space and no hands-on experience? Can a paramedic who lacks the skills for doing so perform a complex physical procedure such as a surgical coniotomy under the guidance of a remote specialist? Task complexity will in the case of co-operative problem solving not only depend on the individuals' skills and knowledge, but also on the capability to transfer the skills and knowledge in real-time to the other person.

The importance of involving the broader social and organisational context, becomes quite clear when we consider the fact that, for example, the ambulance nurse has to know in the first place where to find which expertise, that he has to be able to reach the physician, who should be available at that moment for delivering immediate support, that available resources and subsequent actions have to be taken into account and planned collectively, etc. This new work situation will set new requirements to the organisation of medical emergency care and the information-related and social relations that have to be established between the actors involved. Here, we can expect differences in perceived usefulness between the different actors, as well as conflicts between the usefulness that the individual actors experience as opposed to the costs/benefits for the organisation as a whole. Also, conflicts between performance criteria and the more personal criteria - such as career opportunities, developments of knowledge and skills, workload, autonomy, task variety etc. - have to be taken into account.

A Closer Look at Emergency Medicine

Co-operative or distributed problem solving and decision making introduces special problems and sets new requirements to modelling work (see for an overview Rasmussen *et al.*, 1991). The usefulness of the application outlined above for emergency medicine as a whole, no longer depends only on the individual tasks to be performed (e.g. by the ambulance paramedic, and the hospital physician). Within emergency medicine several actors are involved in co-ordinating their activities with the common objective of patient treatment. As the usefulness of mobile multimedia communications will depend on the affordances and barriers it introduces to the collective organisation of work activities, the individual is no longer the unit of analysis. Task analysis, in terms of individual tasks and subtasks and the required senso-motoric and cognitive processes (see e.g. Kirwan and Ainsworth, 1992), needs to be supplemented with the analysis of social and organisational aspects of work. To cover these aspects, contextual approaches are needed to model the collective performance of tasks.

Promising approaches to studying context are based on activity theory (Nardi, 1996a), situated action models (Suchman, 1987) and the notion of distributed cognition (Hutchins, 1991, 1994) (see for a comparison Nardi, 1996b). Very useful for uncovering the informal, i.e. the actual versus prescribed, aspects of work, as well as the details of activities, tool use and the physical working environment, is interactive field observation or anthropological/ ethnographic research (e.g. Hughes *et al.*, 1993). A good example of a method that makes the ethnographic approach more cost and time efficient, with a clear focus on the redesign of current work practice, is the contextual inquiry and design approach of Holtzblatt and Beyer (1996). Similar to their approach we have built three work models of emergency medicine. Based on several sources (job and work process descriptions, professional journals, field observations, workplace visits and interviews) the actors involved are identified and an analysis is made of their roles, tasks and activities, as well as the communication and co-ordination processes between them. Besides the information-related aspects, the social relations between the actors, and the organisational and cultural context is analysed. The analysis results in several representations showing the workflow, context and sequence of work activities. Together, the three models offer a reference framework for the development of scenarios and for guiding the assessment of the consequences of the new way of working sketched in the scenarios.

Workflow

In the workflow model (part of which is shown in figure 11.4) a representation is given of the actors, their roles and the communication and co-ordination between them. The actors involved in the process of emergency medicine are the despatch centre, ambulance services, the hospital physicians, the emergency/ first aid department, the mobile medical team (in special circumstances), as well as general practitioners, the police, fire-brigades, the patient(s) and bystanders.

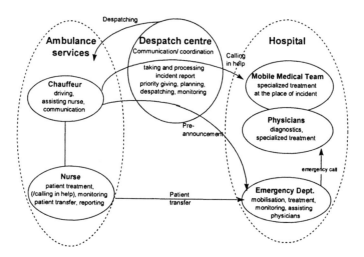

Figure 11.4 Part of the workflow model: actors, their roles and communication between them

The ambulance services are called in at the moment the incident report has been processed by the dispatch centre, which is the central co-ordination and communication unit. One of the available ambulances is sent to the place of incident, where the ambulance nurse, assisted by the chauffeur, delivers first aid to the victim[1]. When required, more ambulances and/or the mobile medical team are called in (before or after arrival of the first ambulance). This, as well as the planning of resources and the pre-announcement to the hospital, is done by the despatch centre. If necessary, the emergency department calls in a team of

---

[1] The chauffeurs' training is comparable to that of a basic Emergency Medical Technician in the US situation. The nurse has a diploma in basic nursing, intensive care and coronary care. After high school nurses get an average training of 7 years.

specialised hospital physicians for further treatment[2]. Specific patient data are in most cases transferred to the hospital nurses and/or physicians at the moment of arrival at the emergency department.

Context

The role of the despatch centre as the central co-ordinator is also expressed in the context model, part of which is shown below. In this model, the organisational rules and criteria, and social relations in terms of interests and (potential) conflicts, expectancies and attitudes towards each other are represented. The model is focused on the application of direct remote expert support and can serve as an artefact for discussion with the potential user community about the consequences of the application for their roles in the process. For example, the aspect of 'keeping the role of central co-ordination and communication centre' and the actual involvement of the despatch centre in the evaluation process as a non-user of mobile multimedia communications, turned out to have important consequences for the joint redesign of the situation outlined in the scenario.

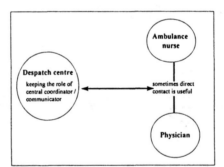

Figure 11.5 An example of interests and potential conflicts between actors

Sequence of Work Activities

The process of emergency medical care actually starts before the first call to the despatch centre. In some cases first aid is delivered by the bystanders, the general practitioner, or the other emergency services (police, fire-brigade), as is shown in the flow of work activities in figure 11.6. It is crucial that the ambulance service is called immediately and that they

---

[2] In the Netherlands there are no emergency physicians or specialists in accident and emergency medicine. The surgeon is in charge of the emergency department. When needed, another specialist like an anesthesiologist, neurologist and/or a cardiologist is called in.

arrive as quickly as possible. The first hour from the time of incident/accident is of vital importance to the patient. Within this hour the patient has to be treated on the basis of assessment and priorities. Essential to pre-hospital medical care is treatment based on the fast and accurate assessment of symptoms and priorities rather then on a detailed anamnesis and diagnosis, as is the case in the in-hospital care. Paramount is the identification of disorders related to the airway (A), breathing (B), circulation (C), and disability or dysfunctioning of the central nervous system (D). Assessment and treatment of injured patients is protocolised according to the ABCD action procedure developed for the Pre Hospital Trauma Life Support (PHTLS). The urgent and physical, action-oriented nature of emergency medicine sets the stage for the evaluation of a work scenario in which the ambulance and hospital work activities are synchronised through mobile multimedia communications. In the current situation it is only after the decision for a specific hospital, patient transport and transfer, that the responsibility for further diagnostics and treatment is carried over to the hospital specialists and nurses at the emergency department.

The work sequence model is directly used for the development of the future work scenario. To develop a rich and realistic picture of future working practice the sequence model also represents the concrete actions performed, besides the representation of the more general activities shown in figure 11.6. An example of the actions performed in the activity of assessing the patient's state is follows:

- ambulance nurse introduces him/herself
- assessment of the level of consciousness on the basis of the patient's reaction, checks pupils
- checks the airway, frequency and depth of breathing, skin color, saturation, pulse, blood pressure, bleeding, pain
- asks for information from the patient/ bystanders
- chauffeur connects heart monitor, makes ECG
- assessment of heart rhythm

Besides the actions and activities performed and the social and organisational setting, as modelled below, the physical environment (e.g. noise, light, mobility etc.) will play an important role in the contribution that mobile multimedia communications can make to emergency medicine. Because the actors are physically dispersed and may have a changing working environment because of their mobility, multiple physical environments have to be taken into account (hospital wards, radio room, ambulance, helicopter, people's homes, out on the street).

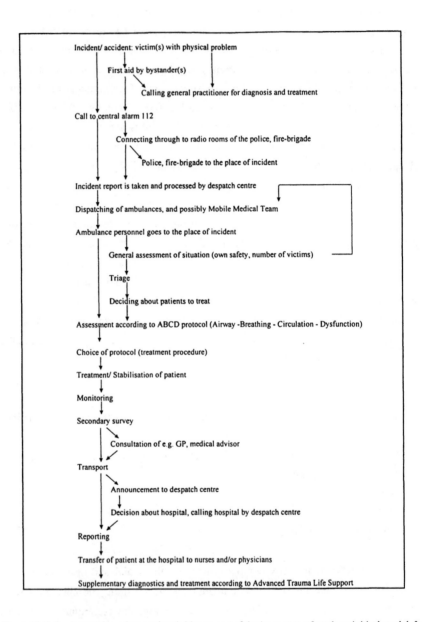

Figure 11.6 Representation of general activities as part of the 'sequence of work activities' model. In practice activities are often performed in parallel.

The Future Work Scenario

A key problem to the design of new technologies and work is communicating the technological (im)possibilities to the workers on the one side and communicating the work context to the developers on the other side. Especially in the case of future technologies such as mobile multimedia communications, it is hard for the workers to formulate their needs and the problems and risks introduced by the new technology, or even to imagine what the technology could mean for their future work. Therefore, to involve the potential user community in the design and evaluation process as experts on their work, a representation of future work activities supported by the new technology is required. Envisioning of future work will allow us to transcend the immediate needs and requirements that are apparent in the current working practice.

A good medium to represent and analyse how a new technological system might impact on its users' work activities are usage scenarios. These comprise a vocabulary that is rich and accessible to the potential users (as well as developers), so that they can help to define the technology and the problems it introduces. The focus is not on the technology as such, but rather on the use of the technology in concrete, daily work activities. This focus contrasts with the established view on system development (see figure 11.7).

The scenario perspective:	*The establishment view:*
concrete descriptions	abstract descriptions
focus on particular instances	focus on generic types
work driven	technology driven
open-ended, fragmentary	complete, exhaustive
informal, rough, colloquial	formal, rigorous
envisioned outcomes	specified outcomes

Figure 11.7 from Carroll (1995)

The work scenario we have developed for emergency medicine presents a narrative, film-like description of the envisioned use of mobile multimedia communications in the daily work activities of and communication between those involved in incident/accident handling. It is meant to direct the thought and discussion processes of the potential user community in a concrete and contextual way. Our approach differs from other scenario-based approaches (see Carroll, 1995) which focus on individual human-computer interaction and user interface design. The successful introduction of communication technologies and systems for computer supported co-operative work is much more dependent on the ability to assess and plan the social and organisational implications of the systems than do other forms of computer systems (Eason and Olphert, 1996; Arnold and Van den Anker, 1997). The application of mobile multimedia communications may change the roles of the potential users in the work process, as well as the allocation of tasks, responsibilities and procedures. The scenarios' focus on the new organisation of collective work activities and communication patterns should enable the assessment of the system's impact on these social and organisational aspects.

The scenario approach focuses on particular cases taken from daily working practice that are worked out in detail. This may require additional analysis of the current situation, by techniques such as field observation, conversation analysis (see Greatbatch *et al.*, 1995), or simulation and/or cognitive walkthrough of particular cases. Because only a few work situations can be worked out in detail in the work scenario, the selection of input variables for these situations is important. In our study we used the following input criteria:
1) complex problem solving situations, 2) representation of all potential users in different settings, 3) variation in user expertise and type of multimedia communications, 4) task representativeness. On the basis of this input one or more futuristic incident/accident handling stories are worked out.

1) complex situations, in which remote support, e.g. from physicians to ambulance personnel, can be useful; the situations selected were a trauma and a complex reanimation case;

2) various users and non-users are presented in various physical settings (e.g. a cardiologist from the hospital as well as a trauma physician from the trauma helicopter);

3) variation in expertise and in the type of multimedia communications. Audio/ speech, physiological data, still and moving video images are used to support the various activities and levels of expertise involved. To cover the different kinds of expertise, not only communication between the ambulance nurse and physician was worked out within the trauma scenario, but also the remote support from an ambulance nurse to the police, who often arrive earlier at the place of incident. Because of the differences in expert-expert versus expert-non-expert dialogues (see Falzon, 1991), different contributions of mobile multimedia communications may be expected in these two cases.

4) the scenarios must represent the most important activities as shown in figure 11.6: co-ordination activities, diagnosis, decision making, physical task performance.

SCENE 13   EXTERIOR   PLACE OF INCIDENT   DAY

The chauffeur passes the syringe to the nurse who injects the propofol. The ambulance nurse resumes the intubation. He inserts the tube, and checks its position. He takes his stethoscope and listens to the breath sounds. He moves the tube a little bit and auscultates again. He fixes the tube, and takes the stethoscope. We hear the patient's breathing through the stethoscope. The patient is ventilated by using a bag-valve-mask resuscitator. The nurse pushes the button for audio contact with the trauma helicopter.

> NURSE
>
> Absent breath at the left side of the thorax, less movement.
>
> Could be a pneumothorax. How long will it take you to get here?

> PHYSICIAN
>
> At least five minutes. Please percuss the thorax.

> NURSE
>
> *(while percussing)*
>
> Left hyperresonance to percussion.

> PHYSICIAN
>
> O.k. pneumothorax.

> NURSE
>
> Condition gets worse. I have to do a puncture now.

> PHYSICIAN
>
> O.k. we will monitor it.

SCENE 14   INTERIOR   HELICOPTER

The trauma physician activates moving video on his screen.

We see the nurse at the location of the accident getting a thick intravenous cannulas.

> PHYSICIAN
>
> *(to nurse)*
>
> Insert the needle past the upper edge of the rib

We see the nurse moving the needle in the direction of the chest of the casualty.

> PHYSICIAN
>
> A little bit more to the left

The nurse is moving the needle to the left

> PHYSICIAN
>
> A bit more. Hold it! Right, now you can insert the needle.

The nurse is performing the puncture

> NURSE
>
> Air is escaping

Figure 11.8   Two scenes from the trauma scenario, in which the ambulance nurse is performing a puncture because of a pneumothorax, which is not done on a daily basis by the ambulance nurse. During this procedure he is guided by the physician from the trauma helicopter, because immediate action is necessary. The entire emergency medicine scenario comprises 18 scenes and 12 pages

Scenarios can be represented through different media, for example text, process diagrams, drawings, storyboards, mock-ups, scripted prototypes. Even video recordings of current working practice can be used to reflect on design (Suchman and Trigg, 1991; Brun-Cottan and Wall, 1995), but developing video clips of future work is quite a costly way to present a future scenario and is mostly done for marketing purposes. Although less costly, it also takes a considerable amount of time - approximately 2 weeks - to make a detailed textual description of future work activities. Scenarios can be developed at different levels of detail and contextual richness. However, to offer the potential user community a rich framework for the assessment of the usefulness of the new technology for their work activities, the scenario needs to give a realistic description of the concrete actions, physiological parameters, and in our case the evolvement of the co-operative problem solving process, the dialogues, the jargon used, etc. The scenario we developed has the form of a rich, text-based narrative representing concrete settings, events, actions and communication (see Figure 11.8). It is based on a screen-play structure, to provide the liveliness, contextual richness and level of detail required to identify the problems introduced to daily work and interaction.

Evaluation of Future Work

The usefulness of mobile multimedia communications depends on the consequences of the new way of working, in terms of its contribution to the efficiency, effectiveness and safety of task performance and the costs and preconditions involved in realising the envisioned scenario. The problems identified with respect to the scenario can be used for changing the scenario - in terms of the actors, their roles, the users and the activities to be supported by mobile multimedia communications. This should set the stage for eliciting the requirements for the design of useful systems that contribute to safety as well as efficiency and quality of work.

The emergency medicine scenario has been evaluated through workshops, in which ambulance nurses and chauffeurs, hospital physicians, nurses from the hospital emergency department and despatch centre co-ordinators participated. Workshops offer the advantage of group dynamics and discussions during the process of problem analysis. Different from the concept of future workshops (Jungk and Müllert, 1996; Kensing and Madsen, 1991), the thinking and brainstorming of the participants is clearly structured around the future scenario, i.e. the application of the specific technology to their work. Two workshops were organised in two different cities (Utrecht and Rotterdam), lasting 3 to 4 hours, with a maximum of ten participants. After reading the scenario together and an individual brainstorm on opportunities and problems with respect to the scenario, cards are stuck on wall charts, clarified by the participants individually, and subsequently discussed, categorised and integrated by the group. The resulting problem model forms the basis for group work on overcoming the problems by adjusting the scenario.

The advantages that were identified - time profit and the opportunity for higher quality of patient care, i.e. better assessment and decision making in an early stage and more opportunities for early treatment- will depend on the new problems and risks introduced and the possibility of overcoming these by proper design. The problems and requirements identified show the interplay between technology (including the user interface, tools and equipment), people (their roles, knowledge and skills, information needs, privacy and autonomy) and their working context (communication/ co-ordination, and the organisational as well as physical environment), e.g.:

- *technology and expertise:* remote expertise through mobile multimedia communications may create a dependency on support. Therefore, the technical connection should be reliable and without disturbances. The knowledge and skills of the people on the spot must be adequate in case the technology fails, and the availability of the system should not be a reason to take on people who are less educated or experienced. It was indicated that the scenario puts higher demands on the workers' skills in terms of communication abilities. Also, new requirements to the senso-motoric skills should be taken into account in the case of physically performing a complex procedure like a puncture. In particular, the scenario of remote support to the police was found too risky in one of the workshops, unless they had been trained extensively.

- *physical environment, user interface and information needs*: the need for very fast computer interaction was expressed, which could mean a wearable and hands-free computer at the place of incident, e.g. a head mounted display with camera, to enable freedom of movement while communicating. The information the remote physician gets for his diagnosis will be based on a far from ideal video recording situation. Apart from a limited view on the 'problem space', outside light conditions may create problems for the remote physician to see, for example, colour nuances. Interference can be expected between the physical environment and communications through different modalities, e.g. noise at the place of incident, or the sirens of the ambulance interfering with verbal communication and audio information like stethoscope sounds, or, for the ambulance nurse, video on the display that interferes with observing the patient. This led the participants to pose the question of reliability of information that the physician will get for his diagnosis and, as a consequence for the ambulance nurse, the reliability of the diagnosis upon which to act. Also, the switching on and off of the video connection in the scenario was considered to be too dangerous: the physician should be able to monitor the whole process and be able to respond immediately when a deviation is observed.

- *tasks, task division, organisation and responsibility*: the requirement of immediate delivery of remote support can interfere with other, primary tasks, which may lead to task overload. In the scenarios the physicians have to be available for immediate support at any time. This will increase complexity and will put high demands on the organisation of co-operation, e.g. arranging the accessibility and availability of physicians.   Also, the change of the situation to real-time collaborative task performance bears the risk of dividing up the functions of perceiving, thinking, and acting. The physician has to make a diagnosis without hands-on experience, and the ambulance nurse has to act on the basis of limited knowledge and skills. This caused the participants to ask themselves who does what, and who is reponsible for the outcomes. This should be clearly settled by procedures. Also, it was indicated that this situation could reduce the autonomy of the ambulance nurse, who may become a 'robot' that fulfills orders, posing the question of who is in control.

A New Scenario

The scenario focused on the contribution of multimedia communications to the treatment of individual patients, although co-ordination activities by the despatch centre were outlined in the scenario. However, during the workshops a clear role of mobile multimedia was identified for co-ordination (e.g. despatching) and assessment activities (general assessment, triage) earlier in the process of emergency response (see figure 11.6). The workshops participants from the despatch centre indicated that mobile multimedia communications would be useful for an overview of the place of incident to support the general assessment of the situation on the spot and the decision processes with respect to despatching (the number of ambulances, the mobile medical team), triage activities, and deciding about the hospital to which the patient(s) should be transported.

To overcome the above-mentioned problems of interference of mobile multimedia communications with other tasks and the physical environment, and the increase in complexity of the organisation of the new situation, the option of a central expertise centre for the delivery of remote support was worked out. This resulted in a new scenario in which the despatch centre uses mobile multimedia communications for co-ordination activities early in the process of incident handling - e.g. for assessing the situation and despatching - and in which all remote support through mobile multimedia communications is delivered by the expertise centre.

Scenario Usage

The usefulness of the future work scenario itself depends on the processes of scenario construction and evaluation. The main issue in writing the scenario is to represent future work activities and communications in a concrete and realistic way. One part of the scenario was criticised by the workshop participants for being too simplistic. The co-operative problem solving process outlined in this part of the scenario contained very little consultation and conflict, i.e. the complex problem was solved easily when the help of the hospital specialist was called in. As conflict is the essence of screenwriting or narrative film (Blacker, 1986; Field, 1994), the same seems to count for the future work scenario. Realistic narratives of future working practice can be constructed by taking problem cases from the current working practice and translating the actions and communications taking place in the current working practice to the future work situation, as has been done in a later case study on field service engineering.

The process of scenario-based evaluation was positively rated by the workshop participants. They indicated that the scenarios had an important contribution to their ideas about the opportunities and limitations of mobile multimedia communications. Also, during the group evaluation many references were made to the activities that were represented in the scenarios. Some of the participants indicated that the workshop focused too much on the scenarios and that more time should have been available for free discussion. Also, the duration of the workshops was too short for group work on overcoming the identified problems by adjusting the scenario.

OPPORTUNITIES, LIMITATIONS AND FUTURE DIRECTIONS

Scenario usage helps to scope the development area by "setting boundaries around the problem space and the solution space" (McGraw and Harbison,1997). The scenario-based evaluation method outlined above has indeed been useful for the early identification of problems and the exploration of socio-technical requirements of working with mobile multimedia communications. A contextual approach was taken by involving the different emergency medicine actors and their daily working activities in the development, presentation and evaluation of the future scenario. As has just been indicated, this led to the readjustment of the 'design space' outlined in the scenario in terms of the actors, activities, social and physical settings for which the design of the system would be most worthwhile, as a first step in the development process.

However, the contextual information generated by the potential user community is fairly high-level. For design purposes the identified problems, opportunities and requirements still need to be specified, and further analysis is needed on the effects of the new system on efficiency (e.g. exact time profit), safety (the types of errors that are prevented and introduced), effectiveness (quality of patient treatment) and the costs involved in realising the scenarios (e.g. in terms of work load, training, and adjusting policy and procedures). For example, what will be the exact profit, in terms of time and the amount and kind of errors that can be prevented, by the usage scenario shown in figure 11.8, in which a puncture is performed by a person who is insufficiently skilled? Which new risks and errors will be introduced by this scenario and what is the minimum level of skill required?

Moreover, the information generated by the potential user community in the process of early evaluation is not always consistent. There was no clear agreement on the usefulness of some usage situations that were sketched in the scenario. For example, some disagreement arose about the usefulness of the parts in the scenario in which complex procedures are performed at the place of incident by people who lack the necessary skills. The part of the scenario in which a police officer delivers first aid under the remote guidance of an ambulance nurse was indicated by some as too risky and putting too high demands on training and education to make it worthwhile to realise. However, such a scenario needs additional analysis with regard to its consequences on task performance (risks and errors, quality of diagnosis and treatment, time).

Instead of being used as a stand-alone approach, the scenario-based method might be considered especially useful for the early identification of problems and opportunities and the elicitation of preliminary requirements, to be supplemented by other methods for requirement specification and validation and measuring performance. Special attention should be paid to the reliability of the information generated by the potential user community. Users may not have a clear idea about the specific risks and problems introduced, and their needs and requirements, particularly with regard to future technology and work. Early evaluation offers a means of preventing risky and unsuccessful implementations of new systems, but there is great uncertainty with respect to an assessment of the future. Assessment and measurement of the actual consequences of an implemented system on daily work activities is not possible in the case of future technology and work. To narrow the gap between design concepts and evaluation after implementation (see figure 11.7), the future work scenario hypothesizes the influence of preliminary design concepts on daily work activities. In this way the future work scenario offers a contextual tool to support the reflection and discussion process with the objective of identifying usage situations, problems, opportunities and requirements for future technologies and work in an early stage of development.

However, the scenario-based approach is limited to reflection and discussion without any real interaction with the future situation. As our fundamental way of being and learning is actual involvement and not detached reflection, the uncertainty with respect to the consequences for future working practice could be further reduced by more interactive methods to evaluation and design (see also Greenbaum and Kyng, 1991). In our case, the evaluation of the future work scenario and the resulting adjusted scenario served as input for a future work simulation, in which the involved actors play their new roles in the envisioned organisational structure, supported by some mock-up of the future technology. An important direction for future research could be a comparison between the influence of simulations and text scenarios on the evaluation process and outcomes, i.e. the knowledge generated by the different stakeholders, as well as a comparison with more objective and quantitative measures.

REFERENCES

Arnold, A. G. and F. W. G. van den Anker (1997). Evaluation Methodology Telematics Systems: Quality for Users and Context. *SIGCHI Bulletin,* **29,** 72-76.

Blacker, I. R. (1986). *The elements of screenwriting.* Macmillan, New York.

Brun-Cottan, F. and P. Wall (1995). Using video to re-present the user. *Communications of the ACM,* **38** *(5),* Special issue "requirements gathering: the human factor, edited by K. Holtzblatt and H. Beyer.

Carroll, J. M. (ed.) (1995). *Scenario-based design. Envisioning work and technology in system development.* Wiley and Sons, New York.

Eason, K., S. Harker and W. Olphert (1996). Representing socio-technical systems options in the development of new forms of work organization. In: The introduction of information and communication technology (ICT) in organizations (P. Herriot, J.H.E. Andriessen and P.L. Koopman, eds.), *European Journal of Work and Organizational Psychology,* **5** (3), 399-420.

Eason, K. and W. Olphert (1996). Early evaluation of the organisational implications of CSCW systems. In: *CSCW Requirements and evaluation* (P.J. Thomas, ed.), Springer-Verlag, London.

Falzon, P. (1991). Cooperative dialogues. In: *Distributed decision making. Cognitive models for cooperative work* (J. Rasmussen, B. Brehmer and J. Leplat, eds.), Wiley and Sons, Chichester, UK.

Field, S. (1994). *Screenplay. The foundations of screenwriting.* Dell Trade, New York.

Finkelstein, A. (1995). *Report of the Inquiry into the London Ambulance Service. International workshop on software specification and design case study.* Electronic version of the original report, http://www.cs.ucl.ac.uk/staff/A.Finkelstein/las.html.

Gale, S. (1990). Human aspects of interactive multimedia communication. *Interacting with computers*, 2(2),175-189.

Greatbatch, D., C. Heath, P. Luff and P. Campion (1995). Conversation analysis: human-computer interaction and the general practice consultation. In: *Perspectives on HCI: Diverse Approaches* (A. F. Monk and N. Gilbert, eds.), Academic Press, London.

Greenbaum, J. and M. Kyng (eds.) (1991). *Design at work. Cooperative design of computer systems.* Lawrence Erlbaum, Hillsdale, NJ.

Hacker, W. (1986). *Arbeitspsychologie - Psychische Regulation von Arbeitstätigkeiten,* VEB Deutscher Verlag der Wissenschaften, Berlin.

Holtzblatt, K. and H. Beyer (1996). Contextual design: principles and practice. In: *Field methods casebook for software design* (D. Wixon and J. Ramey, eds.), Wiley and Sons, New York.

Hughes, J. A., D. Randall and D. Shapiro (1993). From ethnographic record to system design. Some experiences from the field. *Computer Supported Cooperative Work (CSCW),* 1, 123-141.

Hutchins, E. (1991). The social organization of distributed cognition. In: *Perspectives on socially shared cognition* (L. Resnick, ed.), American Psychological association, Washington, DC.

Hutchins, E. (1994). *Cognition in the wild.* MIT Press, Cambridge, MA.

Jungk, R. and N. Müllert (1987). *Future workshops: how to create desirable futures.* Institute for Social Inventions, London.

Kensing, F. and K. H. Madsen (1991). Generating visions: future workshops and metaphorical design. In: *Design at work. Cooperative design of computer systems* (Greenbaum, J. and M. Kyng, eds.), Lawrence Erlbaum, Hillsdale, NJ.

Kirwan, B. and L. K. Ainsworth (1992). *A guide to task analysis.* Taylor and Francis, London.

McGraw, K. and K. Harbison (1997). *User-centered requirements. The scenario-based engineering process.* Lawrence Erlbaum, Mahwah, New Jersey.

Nardi, B. (Ed.) (1996a). *Context and consciousness: activity theory and human-computer interaction.* MIT Press, Cambridge.

Nardi, B. (1996b). Studying context: a comparison of activity theory, situated action models, and distributed cognition. In: *Context and consciousness: activity theory and human-computer interaction* (B. Nardi, ed.). MIT Press, Cambridge.

Nardi, B. A., A. Kuchinsky, S. Whittaker, R. Leichner and H. Schwarz (1996). Video-as-data: technical and social aspects of a collaborative multimedia application. *Computer Supported Cooperative Work,* 4, 73-100.

Rasmussen, J. (1983). Skills, rules, and knowledge; signals, signs and symbols, and other distinctions in human performance models. *IEEE Transactions on Systems, Man and Cybernetics, SMC*-**13**, 257-266.

Rasmussen, J., B. Brehmer and J. Leplat (eds.) (1991). *Distributed decision making. Cognitive models for co-operative work.* Wiley and Sons, Chichester, UK.

Reason, J. (1990). *Human Error*. Cambridge University Press, New York.

Rice, R. E. (1992). Task analyzability, use of new media, and effectiveness: a multi-site exploration of media richness. *Organization Science*, **3** (4), 475-500.

Schuler, D. and A. Namioka (Eds.) (1993). *Participatory design: principles and practice.* Lawrence Erlbaum, Hillsdale, NJ.

Suchman, L. (1987). *Plans and situated actions.*: Cambridge University Press, Cambridge, UK.

Suchman, L. and R. H. Trigg (1991). Understanding practice: video as a medium for reflection and design. In: *Design at work. Cooperative design of computer systems* (J. Greenbaum,. and M. Kyng, eds.), Lawrence Erlbaum, Hillsdale, NJ.

Van den Anker, F. W. G. and A. G. Arnold (1997). Mobile multimedia communication: a task- and user-centered approach to future systems development. In: *Advances in Human Factors/Ergonomics, Proceedings HCI International '97* (M. J. Smith, G. Salvendy and R. J. Koubek, eds.), vol. 2, pp. 651-654. Amsterdam, Elsevier Science Publishing Company, San Francisco, USA.

Van den Anker, F. W. G. and A. G. Arnold (1998). The usefulness of mobile multimedia comunications: a case study. *Displays,* **18** (4), 193-197, 1998.

Wastell, D. G. and C. L. Cooper (1996). Stress and technological innovation: a comparative study of design practices and implementation strategies. In: The introduction of information and communication technology (ICT) in organizations (P. Herriot, J.H.E. Andriessen and P.L. Koopman, eds.). *European Journal of Work and Organizational Psychology,* **5** (3), 377-379.

CHAPTER 12

MINIMISATION OF RISK IN MEDICAL SYSTEMS BY SYSTEM DESIGN FOR SAFETY

Udo Voges, Forschungszentrum Karlsruhe GmbH, Karlsruhe, Germany

INTRODUCTION

Medical devices can be of great help to the user and to the patient, but they are also often associated with a risk, e.g. risk of malfunction or risk of mishandling, risk to the user and/or to the patient. This risk needs to be minimised or, even better, totally eliminated. Several ways exist to achieve this goal, at least partially, system design for safety being one of them.

This chapter explains the risk associated with using medical systems, presents some examples of risk and discusses the potential benefit of using different design rules to achieve a safe medical system. It is primarily concerned with programmable electronic devices. However, the word 'system' is used, rather than 'device', to emphasise that we are concerned with the role of the device in the system of care, as well as the functioning of the device itself.

While in the early years the selection of the right medical person was the main reason for success or failure, nowadays medical systems of ever greater sophistication and complexity are being used, and with them the risks associated with their use increase. The primary purposes of medical systems are to aid the patient (for instance, the pacemaker), to provide the nurse or other persons with information (as in the intensive care units), to give treatment to a patient (for instance, the radiation equipment) or to assist the surgeon and his team during surgery in the operating theatre (for instance, anaesthesia equipment, surgery equipment). But use of these systems not only brings benefits, there is also risk attached: more or less serious accidents happen while using these medical systems. This may be due – at first sight - to wrong handling of the system, poor location of the system, or failures within the system itself. Most often either the user or the whole system is named as the cause of an accident. Looking more closely at the causes, a design error can often be detected, incorporated into the system at the very beginning. Several measures can be taken to reduce the risk associated with medical systems. These include general safety measures as well as system design issues. Before going into detail, it is necessary to define some of the terms used in the following. In the context of this chapter, we will use the following definitions for the terms, which are based on International standards IEC 61508 (IEC, 1997).

Harm is the physical injury or damage to the health of people.

(Sometimes the damage is not restricted to the health of people and financial loss is included.)

Hazard is the potential source of harm.

(E.g. a hazard can be an error in the system itself or a misuse of the system.)

Risk is the combination of the probability of occurrence of harm and the severity of that harm.

(Risk therefore is associated with probability. So in order to minimise the risk, we can lower the probability of the occurrence of the harm or lower the severity of that harm. If the technology involved is complex, risk seems unavoidable. Only a risk reduction, but not risk elimination, is possible. Furthermore, a limitation of the effect of the risk can be anticipated.)

Tolerable risk is the risk which is accepted in a given context based on the current values of society.

(This tolerable level of risk is always changing in the medical field. It differs from person to person and from time to time, from country to country and depends on the health situation of the person concerned.)

Safety is the freedom from unacceptable risk.

(The risk which is beyond the tolerable risk is unacceptable. Safety is the ideal situation, but it is not the total absence of risk.)

System Engineering is the effective application of scientific and engineering efforts to transform an operational need into a defined system configuration through the top-down iterative process of requirements definition, functional analysis, allocation, synthesis, design optimisation, test, and evaluation.

(Good system engineering must be applied during the design and the development of the medical systems.)

Reasonable foreseeable misuse is the use of a product, process or service under conditions or for purposes not intended by the supplier, but which can happen, induced by the product, process or service in combination with, or as a result of, common human behaviour.

(The misuse, whether intended or not, is a large problem, and the dividing line between intended use and misuse is fuzzy. Often the documentation lacks sufficient information on the restriction of intended use. Nevertheless, not every misuse can be prevented. A simple example from everyday life is the use of a knife. Its intended use is, for instance, to cut bread or meat, but it can easily be misused to threaten people or even kill them and this misuse cannot be eliminated. This is a reasonable foreseeable misuse, but it is tolerated. No one would ban knives in general, only in certain situations where the normal use is not possible.)

In the following sections the risk in medical systems will be discussed first. Several examples of accidents and mishandling of medical systems will be given. Reasons and sources for the risk will be explained. Then, methods of analysing the risk and minimising it in the different system development phases will be discussed. Furthermore, the risk will be looked at from the perspective of some system components. Finally, the benefit of using a system approach will be explained.

RISK IN MEDICAL SYSTEMS

With the development of technology, more and more sophisticated technical systems have been introduced into the medical area, not only into the operating theatre and intensive care units, but also into general patient care and even into home care. In the context of this chapter, we will primarily discuss **medical systems** as electrical, electronic or programmable electronic devices, rather than basic mechanical systems. The main emphasis again will be on programmable electronic medical systems, but most aspects mentioned are also true for the other types.

The use of medical systems quite often results in risk to the user or the environment, with the patient being part of the environment (although sometimes he or she is also the user). The tolerable risk level in the medical area is normally higher than in everyday life: patients need to compare the risk of not applying a certain procedure to the risk associated with the procedures. (This applies only to the ill patient, not to the nurse or the doctor.) Several systems analyses, accident analyses and error reports provide evidence of risk and even of severe accidents. Some examples of varying severity are presented in the following (compare for instance Neumann, 1996 and Voges, 1994).

- A video recorder is set to "play" instead of "record". The required documentation of an endoscopic surgery is subsequently lost. If a complication occurs, no follow-up analysis is possible, but there is no direct harm to the patient.
- By intermixing two hoses, an instrument is wrongly connected to the rinsing/sucking device, resulting in wrong handling. If the instrument is tested prior to intraoperative use, the error can immediately be detected. If it is only detected later during surgery, time is lost while the connections are changed. This can be critical if detected while looking for a blood source in an emergency and it may be that the fluid level is raised rather than reduced.

- The user interface screen of a device is partially covered by cables or other equipment; the leading digit number or even an alarm signal lamp is not visible. If the system is, for instance, for insufflation during minimally invasive laparoscopic surgery, too high pressure is applied, resulting in harm to the patient.
- Too many cables are lying on the floor of the operating theatre and also hanging from equipment, with the risk of hindering the nurse, who may stumble and disconnect the system. Different hazards can be envisaged. Depending on which cable is disconnected, a variety of effects on the surgeon, the surgery or the patient are possible.
- The second pole (grounding) for high frequency coagulation is wrongly positioned, resulting in severe burns to the patient.
- A radiation therapy system is erroneously programmed, resulting in overdose and the death of a patient.
- The use of mobile phones in the ICU results in errors in the ICU equipment. These can result in varying levels of harm.
- The system monitoring the patient in the intensive care unit is not able to deal with newly implanted pacemakers, giving frequent alerts to the nurse. After a while, the nurse will not, or not quickly enough, respond to an alarm which might be an important one (cry-wolf effect).
- Heart pacemakers' and defibrillators' interference with other equipment, such as shoplifting gates, can cause disruption in their functioning which may even lead to failure of the device and the death of a patient.

This list could be extended considerably. These things do happen, even in very good hospitals and in good teams, to one extent or another. The reasons for this are manifold, for instance:

- The systems are becoming too complex to handle.
- The systems are badly designed.
- The users are unfamiliar with the system or inadequately trained.
- Similar systems have different user interfaces, leading to misuse.
- Systems are inadequately maintained.
- Systems are not well suited to maintenance.
- Systems break down.
- Systems are not used in the right context or environment.
- Different systems which are not intended to be used together, are connected with each other or used simultaneously.

One case of a medical system causing unintended death of people will be described in more detail (Leveson, 1993). The Therac-25 is a computerised medical electron accelerator used for cancer treatment with radiation. Between the years 1985 and 1987, six major accidents were reported, each involving a massive overdose, resulting in serious injuries and death. The first accidents were not analysed thoroughly, the sequence of events could not be established, and insufficient modifications and safety actions were made, thus allowing the last major event to occur. The final incident was investigated very closely, the sequence of events could be repeated in tests, and the causes were detected.

An operator who was very quick on the keyboard could make corrections and changes to the radiation parameters, which were not allowed but went by unnoticed by the programme. The resulting overdose was not detected by the system because the measuring device was incapable of measuring such a high dose. Some further problems with the system design and the quality assurance management led to the repetition and late acknowledgement of the accidents. By request from the FDA (USA Department of Health and Human Services, Food and Drug Administration), the manufacturer issued a whole set of modifications to achieve a system where these accidents could not occur again.

Some of the lessons which can be learned from the Therac-25 accidents are as follows:

- Quality assurance procedures during system development are very important.
- Good software engineering principles need to be followed.
- The user interface should be user-friendly, but not if safety is compromised.
- FMEA (Failure mode and effect analysis) and FTA (Fault tree analysis) are useful tools.
- Hardware safety devices (like interlocks) should not always be replaced by software.
- Error messages need to reflect the system state and be easily and correctly understandable by the user.
- Visibility of and communication with the patient during treatment is important.
- Documentation (logging) of user input and actually performed treatment is important (especially for tracking errors).
- Simple 'Repeat action' commands should not be possible in case of potential hazards.

As can be seen, the reasons and the underlying cause for the risk are manifold. However, not only patients suffer from the errors: many doctors involved in adverse events may be haunted by memories of the committed errors. Even apparently small hazards can have disastrous effects. Some of the risk is introduced in the late stages of the system life cycle, some in the early system development phases. In the following sections we will discuss how the risk can be reduced by taking different steps during the individual system development phases.

THE DEVELOPMENT PHASES

In this section we will discuss briefly the risk and its occurrence, analysis and elimination in the different system development phases. Without loss of generality, we will restrict the analysis to the basic phases of design, manufacture, use, and maintenance, which can be mapped to every system life cycle with a more detailed set of phases. Test and evaluation activities are always seen as an integral part of each of the above phases and not as separate phases. Generally, a good manufacturing practice, which covers the total life cycle, is a very important issue, involving use of quality assurance management procedures on a high level (cf. FDA, 1995).

Design

The design phase is probably the most important phase for minimising risk because it is the initiating phase. The requirements analysis needs to clarify the basic purpose of the system, the intended function and operation, and its use. The environment in which the system will be used is described and documented. The agreement between the user and the manufacturer on these descriptions and documents on the requirements is very important, since they form the basic set of information for the later stages. Not only the basic functional requirements need to be assessed, but also - from the safety point of view most importantly - the safety-critical ones. Since some of the requirements may contradict each other to some degree or require different solutions, a weighting process is necessary to see which of the requirements are most important (Tsai, 1998). Here the safety-criticality is an important aspect.

First of all, a thorough risk analysis is necessary in order to identify all the possible risks associated with the system under consideration. For each risk the probability of its occurrence, the consequence in the sense of damage and the probable reasons for its occurrence need to be given. Each risk identified then needs to be associated with a plan to eliminate or reduce this risk. Wherever possible, this should result in the elimination of the risk in the design phase. This can be achieved by, for example, selecting special components, including redundancies and diversity, and even by installing an extra safety system. A clear distinction is necessary between the parts which are to be realised in hardware, and those which are implemented in software. Safety shall not be sacrificed to beauty; a simple user interface is not always the safest solution. Design is the phase where the most can be achieved concerning safety.

The risk analysis has to look not only at the overall design of the system, but also the individual components need to be analysed. Both obvious and frequent events need to be inspected, but the improbable events need to be taken into account too. A generally improbable event can have higher probability due to unskilled users, unfortunate circumstances or unusual environment. In case existing components are reused, the related existing risk analysis needs to be inspected and reviewed and the risk of reusing components needs to be considered. As an example, in the Ariadne-5 rocket system some software from the Ariadne-4 was reused without careful enough rechecking of all required constraints. The result was the expensive failure of the maiden flight of Ariadne-5. This is not to say that reuse of components is wrong. Generally it is a good practice to reuse proven parts, especially software, but sufficient care is necessary to check the reusability and the interfaces.

Besides the risk analysis, the construction work on a structured design is important. The modularisation of the system influences not only the implementation and manufacturing of the system, but also its subsequent use and maintenance. The positive influence of modularisation can lead to a risk reduction in the use of the system.

Manufacture

The risk analysis mentioned above concerning the final product can also be applied to the system development process itself, leading to the identification of risks and associated counter measures. Then, within each phase, quality assurance needs to check that the appropriate counter measures have been installed. This is not only true for the manufacturing phase, but also to some extent to the other phases (FDA 1995).

The risk associated with the manufacturing phase itself is most often the smallest one if said manufacturing procedures are in place. Standard quality assurance procedures attempt to guarantee that a product of best quality will be the result of the manufacturing phase, starting with the selection of appropriate material.

During and at the end of the manufacturing process, extensive tests by the development team and in addition by a representative selection of the user population are necessary. The use and the usability of the system must be analysed very closely in order to detect possible risks and misuse. Verification of the system, in the sense of checking that the system is correct, is necessary and also validation, i.e. that the correct system has been developed, are important.

Use

While the potential for risk is most often laid in the early phases of system development, any malfunctioning will show up during the 'use' phase. The two main categories are failure of the system itself and mishandling by users.

The risk due to system failure can largely be overcome by:

- System design: Internal failures must be detected by some form of redundancy. Failures should be tolerated because of additional internal checks, leading to a fail-safe behaviour. However, this is something which needs to be attempted during the design phase. It is too late to do something in the use phase.
- Quality assurance: Selection of good quality material and personnel, together with sufficient validation and verification activities, should result in a high quality product with low failure probability. This is to be taken account of during manufacturing the system.

The occurrence of mishandling or misuse of the system can be reduced by:

- having a good overall system design
- having a good user interface
- making sure that only the right people (the correctly trained people) use the system.

While the first two are problems of the design phase, the last one has to be dealt with in the use phase. The training of the user is a necessary and important aspect. Regulations always state that only trained people are allowed to use and apply medical devices. Training is simplified if different devices have identical interfaces and use patterns in order to maintain consistency. Training is aided by a good system and user interface design, reinforcing the importance of the design phase.

Maintenance

Maintenance of the system is an important issue in order to keep it in good working order. While on the one hand the saying is "never touch a (good) running system" - do not change or modify it - some checks are necessary at certain time intervals to keep the system running, detect developing risks, assess wear and tear, control reported self-repaired errors etc.

As always, sufficiently trained personnel are necessary for this job, otherwise there will be the risk of introducing errors into the system instead of removing them. This is also a topic for quality assurance. It must be clear who is allowed to do which part of the maintenance, which parts are to be maintained only by the manufacturer, and which ones by the user, where medical personnel can carry out maintenance, and where is it the job of a technician. Nevertheless, the system should not be 'maintained to death'.

Development Process for Non-Medical Systems

In the design of other, non-medical systems, the use of computerised design tools is helping to reduce the risk. For instance, in the design of the Boeing 777, the plane was first completely designed by the use of computers. All measurements were made by simulation tools. This resulted in a shorter life cycle and in fewer design errors, which would have been detected only in the late phases. The safety of the plane was increased and the risk of malfunctioning was reduced.

In the automotive industry, computer simulation is also used for checking the feasibility of maintenance: the assembly and deassembly of the motor and other parts of the automobile are tested in virtual reality, in order to check that all parts which need to be maintained are easily accessible. This is not so much safety oriented, but maintenance costs oriented.

These techniques are also available in the design of medical devices. The use of modelling tools and of virtual reality environments can be helpful in designing the systems themselves and the user interface. They allow an early involvement of the user in checking the design and the usability of the system. Simulation can be used for evaluation of the risks in the system, the fault tolerance and the behaviour in case of errors.

THE SYSTEM COMPONENTS

While all parts of the system can to a different degree incorporate a hazard and be the source of a risk, only the user interface and the system structure, as the two main factors, will be discussed in the following section.

User Interface

Considerable risk is associated with the user. In order to reduce the likelihood of human errors in using a medical system, a careful design of the user interface is necessary. This relates to human engineering, human factors, usability engineering or ergonomics.

There are different ways of dealing with user errors and how to categorise them (compare, for instance, Grams, 1998). Often the user is blamed for the error while in reality the system design is at fault (which may be due to the human error in designing the system). Bad systems, or bad user interfaces, can force the user to commit errors.

There are different aspects to the human interface, as there are different ways a human being can interact with the system. One aspect is the perceived output of the system.

This is, for example,

- the video screen for an endoscopic picture,
- scales for the measurements of pressure, flow, etc.
- digital output for values set by dials,
- control lights for the status
- sound of alarms.

In order to reduce the overall risk, the output must be presented in such a way that it is unambiguous and is always interpreted correctly. In emergency situations it is essential that the output is immediately understood at a quick glance, without lengthy text or the necessity to refer to user manuals.

From the safety point of view, it is most important that the system either functions correctly or, rather than functioning incorrectly, not at all. Fail-safe behaviour is needed, and the safe state which needs to be achieved in case of failure must be made clear. In many systems, the fail-safe state is identical to the stop state, but in others basic functionality is required even in the case of failure. In the case of possible errors, an alarm can alert the users. But the use of the alarms has to be done carefully: too many alarms, especially too many false alarms, can have a negative effect. We will experience the so called cry-wolf effect: the user will stop listening and reacting to an alarm, will ignore it, the alarm becomes useless and will only be a design feature making the licensing authority happy but not the user.

Another aspect is the user input. All aspects of ergonomics and human factors should be looked at. The design of the user interface needs to take into account that the system might not always be handled under perfect conditions:

- The input device can be in a sub-optimal position (too far away, too low / too high, low light, poorly accessible).
- The user is not always trained as he or she should be.
- The user has no time to familiarise him/herself with all the different options and alternatives in the input.

Some examples for design rules which need to be taken into account when designing the system and its user interface include the following:

- It must be clear which text, explanation, pictogram belongs to which light, knob, dial, etc.;
- The meaning of the text, explanation, pictogram etc. should be intuitively clear and the input choices must be distinct;
- The same interpretation should be valid for a set of systems or all systems in the operating theatre, e.g. identical way of turning/switching, use of colours, etc.

Special attention needs to be given to the different background of the users. This relates not only to the different countries, but even within a country the experience and background of the user of the system changes from one hospital to the other.

A hazard can occur either in normal situations, or sometimes only in abnormal, stress or emergency situations. The user interface needs to be designed in such a way that it can be used correctly in all of these situations. In order to familiarise the medical personnel with the medical systems and also train them with the handling of abnormal events, a medical simulation system would be useful which is able to induce errors or unexpected situations and problems into the normal operation. These errors and problems can be system oriented or patient oriented. The simulation system should help to lead to the recognition of errors, avoidance of errors while dealing with unanticipated problems, and handling errors to minimise their effect.

The aim should be not only to educate the medical personnel but to give them a well designed system with which errors can be avoided as much as possible, or at least be detected early enough to limit their consequences. System errors can also be detected by the use of the simulator, leading to a redesign of the system or the user interface. A more detailed discussion of the systematic and careful design of the user interface for medical devices, especially from the point of view of safety, is given by Sawyer (1997), where an extensive list on further literature is also included.

System Structure

The layout of the system and the design of the system structure must reflect the potential for risk. Some design rules for the system structure must be followed. The system should be separated into safety-critical parts and non safety-critical parts. This is also beneficial for the licensing procedure. Much more effort must go into the design of safety-critical parts. On the other hand, by this distinction it is quite often possible to design a safety kernel of small size, whose properties can be verified. Therefore minimisation of a risk can be achieved. The safety kernel does not usually need a normal user interface, again reducing the risks involved.

Several levels of defence should be incorporated into the system in order to capture possible problems and risk developments as early as possible. These levels of defence can be:

- Several margins for controlling a set point are used: a small bandwidth for normal operation, slightly larger bandwidth for warning, a substantially larger one with more serious warning, and a final boundary resulting in shut-down and fail-safe behaviour.
- One error being tolerated and self-repaired (but with notification to the outside), a second error can still be handled, but results in a more serious warning, and a third error leads to final shut-down.

- The input can be checked differently: in the request for input, the limits are displayed, the input is checked against the limits and automatically corrected, with request to acknowledge correction, or the input is rejected and a new input is requested.

The modularisation of the system into clearly separated, distinct parts with clearly defined interfaces is usually the best approach. The interfaces to other systems should follow a standard pattern. Validation of the correct interconnection should be easy.

Other Aspects

A further aspect which requires greater consideration is the electromagnetic interference (EMI) between different components and different systems. Between the years 1979 and 1995, more than one hundred reports on malfunctioning electronic medical devices probably due to electromagnetic interference were reported to the US FDA (Silberberg, 1996). The level of awareness has increased over time, resulting also in new standards and directives (EEC, 1989). Different approaches can be taken to reduce the effect of EMI, including:

- Design of the components for lower radiation.
- Use of better shielding.
- More testing of equipment to EMC (electromagnetic compatibility).
- Restricting the use of some equipment, and the banning of certain devices in certain areas (e.g. no mobile phones in ICUs).

TOTAL SYSTEM APPROACH

Despite the fact that many things have to be dealt with in individual units, a total system approach is very important. The total system includes not only the medical system itself, but also the environment in which it will be used. Therefore, the operating theatre and all the other systems used within it must be included in the analysis, especially in the risk analysis. This means not only the hardware and software, but also the peopleware, the users and the patients. The user group extends to the people being influenced by the system (e.g. the patient), and even to the people carrying out the maintenance (including cleaning, sterilisation). The design of the system needs to take into account a changing and often unknown environment. No false assumptions should be made and all influencing factors need to be checked, not only statically, but dynamically.

Different aspects of fault tolerance should be incorporated, dealing with hardware, software, environment and user faults. The fault tolerance can be implemented on different levels, but the overall effect needs to be evaluated. Too much fault tolerance, or too many safety features on the lower levels, can also be a burden and result in a loss of safety.

The safety of the system should never be neglected, never compromised to functionality. Furthermore, this must be realised at all levels, from top management to the worker. Management structure is part of the development structure and therefore not only responsible for the success of the product development, but also the safety of the product. Time constraints of a development must not result in neglect of safety.

If a completely new technology is incorporated into an application area, special attention needs to be given to the user, the user acceptance, the users' prior history and experience, and the old technology still in the environment. The introduction of the new system needs to be done in a stepwise fashion in order to familiarise the user with the new way of working. This stepwise approach can also result in a redesign of the system, since during use misinterpretations of the user requirements can be detected (Cook, 1996).

Some lessons can be learned from approaches used in other disciplines. At the moment the medical field is still dominated by medical aspects and not by technical ones. If we look at a more technical area like the nuclear field, defined procedures exist on how to design systems, how to ensure the safety of the systems. Standards exist giving guidance on how to design the different parts of a nuclear power plant. The one that is probably most closely related to the medical field concerning the human-machine interaction and the safety aspects is the IEC 60964 on the design for control rooms in nuclear power plants (IEC, 1989).

CONCLUSION

There are several ways of minimising risk in medical systems, some of which have been explained in this chapter. The main point is that a thorough risk analysis is necessary to identify the possible risks of any system and that risks should be minimised or even eliminated during the system design and development.

For the system design of medical systems, more attention needs to be given to the safety aspects than to the functional aspects. While functions are comparatively easy for a designer and user to discuss and are also in the primary interest of the user, the safety issues are at most only generally recognised. Safety is often neglected or only seen as an unnecessary burden, in the worst case only after accidents have occurred. Special effort and knowledge is necessary to design a dependable system which can be operated in a safe way.

REFERENCES

Cook, R. I. (1996). Adapting to New Technology in the Operating Room. *Human Factors*, **38** (4), 593-613.

EEC (1989). Electro-Magnetic Compatibility Directive. European Economic Community, Directive 89/336/EEC.

FDA (1995). Current Good Manufacturing Practice (cGMP) Final Rule. Report U. S. Food and Drug Administration.

IEC (1989). IEC International Standard - Design for control rooms for nuclear power plants. IEC 60964, 1989-03.

IEC (1997). IEC International Standard - Functional safety of electrical / electronic / programmable electronic safety related systems. IEC 61508, Draft 1997.

Grams, T. (1998). Bedienfehler und ihre Ursachen (Operator Errors and their Causes - in German). *atp,* **40** (3), 53-56, and **40** (4), 55-60.

Leveson, N. G. and C. S. Turner (1993). An Investigation of the Therac-25 Accidents. *IEEE Computer*, **26** (7), 18-41.

Neumann, P. G. (1996). Risks to the Public in Computers and Related Systems. *ACM Software Engineering Notes,* **21** (5), 18ff.

Sawyer, D. (1997). Do It By Design - An Introduction to Human Factors in Medical Devices. Report U. S. Food and Drug Administration.

Silberberg, J.L. (1996). What Can/Should We Learn from Reports of Medical Device Electromagnetic Interference. *Compliance Engineering*, **XIII**, 4, 41-57.

Tsai, W.-T., R. Mojdehbakhsh and S. Rayadurgam (1998). Capturing Safety-Critical Medical Requirements. *IEEE Computer*, **31** (4), 40-41.

Voges, U. and M. Schmitt (1994). *Ist-Analyse vom Einsatz der minimal invasiven Chirurgie (MIC) im Operationssaal* (Is-analysis of the use of minimally invasive surgery (MIS) in the operating theatre - in German). Kernforschungszentrum Karlsruhe.

CHAPTER 13

MEDICAL ERROR AND RESPONSIBILITY IN MANAGED HEALTHCARE

Michael Baram, Boston University School of Law, USA

INTRODUCTION

Physicians and other providers of medical services must meet professional standards of care in diagnosing and treating their patients. If they fail to do so by committing medical error injurious to a patient, they are subject to liability for medical malpractice, and may incur reputational damage, loss of hospital privileges, and even decertification. Thus, avoidance of injurious medical error is essential, and causes many physicians to practice 'defensive medicine' by taking costly precautions in treating patients. (Furrow *et al.*, 1997).

Most patients now receive medical services under government or employer-funded healthcare programmes which pay for their medical needs. These programmes manage the delivery of medical services and therefore influence the quality and cost of patient care. To contain costs within programme resource limitations, they impose practice and cost constraints on physician diagnosis, treatment and referral of patients. As public demand for medical services, new technologies, preventive medicine and long term care rises, so do the costs incurred, thereby causing health programme management to impose progressively more stringent controls on physicians. (Sigma, 1998).

Thus, the traditional autonomy of physicians in determining and providing for a patient's medical needs is being progressively reduced. Anecdotal evidence suggests that these circumstances have caused harm to some patients and put many others at increased risk due to inadequate medical attention or medical errors by physicians working under such constraints. Such circumstances also put physicians at increased risk of liability and other adversities. (Rochefort, 1998; Robbins, 1998).

The problem of injurious medical error in the context of managed healthcare therefore requires that attention be given firstly to factors which influence the physician-patient relationship, such as the cost and practice constraints imposed on physicians by healthcare managers and secondly to the risk management programmes they employ.

MEDICAL ERROR

The term 'medical error' is usually used to denote a simple mistake by a physician, such as unintentionally prescribing the wrong drug or dosage for a patient. It also more broadly denotes a physician's failure to meet a professional standard of medical care in diagnosing or treating a patient's condition due to negligence, lack of expertise, or other root cause (such as careless disregard of a patient's symptom or need for referral to a specialist, or performing inferior quality surgery). Thus, the term covers physician determinations, actions or omissions which are unintentionally erroneous or inferior according to professional criteria. (Furrow *et al.*, 1997).

If the medical error causes injury to the patient (such as worsening the patient's condition or causing a new harm), then the physician is held responsible. In the United States, the legal doctrine of medical malpractice (a form of professional negligence) applies to such cases and enables the victim (patient) to recover monetary damages from the physician (or his insurer), unless there is evidence showing that the physician intentionally deviated from the applicable standard of care in treating the patient, that the deviation was medically reasonable, that the physician fully informed the patient, a priori, of the deviation and its possible risks, and that the informed patient gave voluntary consent. Thus, securing a patient's prior informed consent affords protection from liability to the physician who intentionally provides a reasonable form of treatment which does not meet conventional practice (as in cases where conventional practice has low probability of defeating a patient's terminal illness, or would put an aged or infirm patient at additional risk or extreme discomfort).

Thus, the standard of care for the patient is the key criterion for determining if a physician has committed medical error and informed consent serves as a safeguard for patients against unacceptable deviations and for physicians against liability. Both concepts have been at issue in numerous lawsuits in the United States for decades and have been calibrated by the courts to meet new circumstances. For example, as communications have improved, the standard of care, once based on local medical practice or custom, is now usually based on generic or national standards of medical practice (especially for medical specialties), as provided by medical treatises and other 'mainstream' medical indicia. Similarly, finding that physicians often minimise risks in seeking informed consent, the courts have held that informed consent requires that physicians more fully inform patients of risks and other potential consequences that a reasonable person would want to know.

However, the courts have not been as responsive to change in deciding medical malpractice cases in which new health programme constraints imposed on physicians contributed to malpractice such as the commission of injurious medical error. (Leitner, 1997). In only a few cases have courts held healthcare programmes and hospitals liable for such harms when the physicians involved have been employees of such organisations, under legal doctrines of corporate negligence or an employer's vicarious liability for negligent acts by its employees.

The vast majority of physicians work as independent contractors to such healthcare programmes. Although contractually obligated to provide services in compliance with the programme's practice guidelines and cost constraints, independent practitioners continue to be held fully responsible by the courts for injurious outcomes if they failed to meet applicable standards of care in treating their patients. Thus, courts in most cases of injurious medical error do not recognise organisational culpability and persist in maintaining that the independent contractor physician be held responsible and liable for sub-standard treatment irrespective of cost considerations and the physician's obligations to 'third parties' (such as the healthcare programme he serves) (Stoeckl, 1998).

American law governing claims of injurious medical error therefore continues to support the 'moral covenant between physician and patient' that derives from the Hippocratic Oath, which characterises medicine as an esteemed profession of care-giving and exhorts doctors to 'do no harm.' American law also gives relatively free rein to a proliferation of governmental and private employer healthcare programmes and their use of profit-seeking management firms as intermediaries to impose practice and cost constraints on physicians. As a result, healthcare management "as steadily and increasingly attacked the moral centre of the doctor-patient relationship...by interfering with and constraining this relationship...all the while standing back and claiming that they have nothing to do with medical decisions." (Hiepler and Dunn, 1998).

Rising tension between the physician's ethical and legal obligations to the patient to practice medicine in the best professional way and the concurrent legal obligation to comply with the cost and practice constraints contractually-imposed by health programme management has led to many calls for reform. Physicians seeking to regain autonomy, public interest groups seeking national enactment of a 'patient bill of rights' and state legislative moves to hold healthcare management accountable for injurious medical outcomes caused by their physician contractors are among the main reforms now before the American public (USLW, 1998). Given the necessity of healthcare programmes to pay for the medical needs of citizens, and the inevitability of the need for management controls to contain costs, it seems that the most pragmatic solution is to recognise organisational culpability in injurious medical outcomes and allocate responsibility and liability accordingly (Daniels and Sabin, 1998; Bovens, 1998).

"If managed care chooses to impose the many restrictions and constraints on the relationship between doctor and patient that it currently does, then any and all overseers and administrators causing the interference should be held to the same standard as doctors...a high moral and ethical standard ... that...needs to be applied of all participants in the health care delivery system." (Hiepler and Dunn, 1998). If this conflict remains unresolved, health programme managers will face increasing market and public pressures to voluntarily prevent patient risk of medical error more effectively. If it is resolved in the manner suggested above (by making health management legally accountable) health programme managers will face increasing liability and economic losses unless they prevent medical error more effectively. Thus, the most likely alternative scenarios produce the same need for health programmes to implement effective programmes for safeguarding patients from medical error.

HEALTHCARE PROGRAMMES AND MANAGED CARE

Healthcare programmes in developed nations have grown to significant economic proportions, and now comprise more than 10% of gross domestic product in Germany, Switzerland and France. In the United States, publicly-funded and private employer health programmes pay for the medical needs of more than 200 million persons, expend over $1 trillion annually, and account for 14% of gross domestic product (Sigma, 1998).

Although national systems differ in many respects, all must contend with the need to equitably and effectively allocate limited resources for quality care in the face of rising public demand for medical services. In addition to conventional medical services, patients want rapid exploitation of new technologies such as gene therapy and use of sophisticated instrumentation to improve their health status and life expectancy. However, introduction into medical services of advances in genetics, nutrition, the health and behavioural sciences, and biomedical engineering involves considerable investment, maintenance, training and operating costs, and a continuum of follow-on expenditures. For example, new techniques for enhancing human reproductive capabilities often cause premature multiple births which necessitate extensive use of life support systems, developmental treatments and prolonged physical therapy for the newborns. Similarly, growing demand for preventive medicine and long-term care, fields which have no apparent boundaries, is resulting in increasing expenditures.

As a result, greater emphasis is being given to the application of management methods to assure the cost-effectiveness of medical services and cost-containment of health programme expenditures overall. In the United States, this has led to adoption of the 'managed care' concept and the rapid deployment of private managed care organisations (MCOs) to serve as the 'intermediaries' between the healthcare programmes which pay for medical services (the 'payers') and the physicians and hospitals which provide medical services (the 'providers') to persons eligible for such services under the terms of their health programme coverage. Most Americans needing medical services must therefore deal with a veritable 'medical enterprise' of payers, intermediaries and providers who are contractually connected and function in a competitive, cost and profit-driven healthcare marketplace (Sigma, 1998).

A major health insurer's analysis describes the American healthcare system as "a market rife with paradox. The tremendous expenditure of resources produces on the one hand cutting-edge technologies and at its best the highest quality of care available anywhere, yet at the same time does not preclude the exclusion of more than 40 million Americans from the system. It is a market that permits the coexistence of cut-throat competition and gross inefficiency. It simultaneously creates financial incentives for care givers to withhold treatment under the guise of managed care, yet forces them to perform unnecessary tests and procedures to avoid accusations of malpractice." (Sigma, 1998).

Like many other critiques, the analysis targets the implementation of managed care by MCOs "...as managed care organisations (MCOs) penetrate even further into the United States' health care market, many Americans are expressing misgivings over the ability and willingness of these organisations to provide high quality comprehensive health care services. The uneasiness is reinforced by numerous anecdotal accounts of care withheld or restricted by MCOs, often with tragic consequences. A slew of recent state and federal legislation governing the treatment protocols of MCOs gives the appearance of validating these concerns." (Sigma, 1998).

Thus, the management system at the core of the medical enterprise in the United States is being called into question. Do MCOs manage payer funds and provider services in a manner which reduces the quality of medical treatment? Do MCOs take appropriate steps to prevent medical practices from being injurious to patients?

Managed Care as a Source of Patient Risk

MCOs are hired by health programmes to implement the managed care concept, i.e. to assure that programme funds are expended cost-effectively on medical services of requisite quality and that total costs are contained within programme parameters. Since MCOs compete for health programme clients, their financial viability depends on superior performance.

Performance involves contracting physician and hospital providers of the medical services needed by patients covered by the programme in order to establish terms and fees in payment for their work. In negotiating such matters, individual physicians have weak bargaining power and many are now joining physician associations for collective strength in negotiating these contracts. The main purpose of the terms and fees is to control the costs of patient care by limiting the physician's compensation and offering various inducements for the physician to be more cost effective in providing patient care. For example, the contractual arrangement often provides a personal financial incentive in the form of a periodic bonus payment if the physician reduces patient hospitalisations or referrals to specialists below designated levels (Robbins, 1998).

The contract also usually provides for 'capitation', the payment of a fixed sum per month to the physician contractor for all services to be provided for eligible persons, irrespective of the number of patients actually seen or cared for. Physicians accept capitation, despite its potential inadequacy for providing quality care, because it helps to cover basic overhead costs of their practice. Consequently they must then struggle to reduce costs when serving the needs of many patients in order to derive personal income. This, in turn, increases the likelihood of inferior patient care, medical error, malpractice liability, unethical practices towards patients and 'gaming' with MCOs (Robbins, 1998).

In addition, MCOs require that providers follow 'medical practice guidelines' which the MCOs have developed or adopted from other sources (Sisk, 1998). This marks a direct intervention by programme managers into the physician's discretionary use of medical expertise. The practice guidelines serve as templates for physicians to apply in determining and providing for the needs of patients. Each guideline represents a uniform, cost-effective protocol for dealing with a particular medical condition despite the unique features of each patient (Robbins, 1998; Leitner, 1997).

As a result, "many providers feel that they have lost control over the ability to practice medicine and that...intermediaries now control the process...a backlash is beginning to occur as providers seek to reestablish their autonomy and control in the practice of medicine...." (Sigma, 1998). Practice guidelines have also been accused of causing many detriments to healthcare. According to the National Institute of Medicine, which has been enlisted by the federal government to study guideline development: "guidelines have been tied in some way - positively or negatively -to concerns about the quality of care, patient empowerment, professional autonomy, medical liability, access to care, rationing, competition, benefit design, utilization variation, bureaucratic micromanagement of health care, and more." (National Institute of Medicine, 1995).

Despite their criticality for patient care, the practice guidelines imposed on physicians are not subjected to prior official and objective appraisal by disinterested medical or public health boards or members of the public. Thus, they are used without official safeguards and certification regarding their efficacy or the risks they may pose.

The practice guidelines used by MCOs have, in many instances, been voluntarily developed by private medical associations (such as the American Cancer Society, the American Geriatric Association and the American College of Radiology) and public medical organisations (National Cancer Institute, National Institutes of Health, for example). However, not being subject to any official screening, review or coordination procedures, practice guidelines are freely proliferating and multiple guidelines for a particular medical condition are available for MCO selection and adoption (e.g. 35 guidelines for breast cancer screening, treatment, reconstruction, etc.; 15 guidelines for anesthesiology). Thus, when a physician has several patients with the same condition, with each patient covered by a different healthcare programme which has imposed a different practice guideline for this condition on the physician, the physician must treat each patient in accordance with the applicable guideline. As a result, physician treatment varies accordingly among these patients. (American Medical Association, 1998).

In its Directory of Clinical Practice Guidelines, a compendium of some 1900 practice guidelines, the American Medical Association (AMA) cautions that "While it is generally recognized that...practice guidelines may serve as a useful resource, they may not be appropriate for an individual patient. Clinical practice guidelines are an aid to, not a substitute for, professional judgment in addressing individual patient needs."

The AMA plans to establish a pilot programme for evaluating and coordinating practice guidelines, and intends to grant AMA certification to guidelines which are developed and regularly revised by physician organisations on the basis of current professional knowledge, which explicitly describe how they were developed, and which "assist practitioner and patient decisions about appropriate health care for specific clinical circumstances."

Of particular concern are the many practice guidelines used by MCOs which have not been developed by medical or health associations. For these, the AMA merely provides that non-physician organisations (such as MCOs, health insurers, government agencies, etc.) should consult with relevant physician organisations prior to their development and implementation. It also recommends that MCO's accept propositions that physicians "retain autonomy to vary from...guidelines without retribution in order to provide the quality of care that meets the individual needs of their patients" and that "third parties" such as MCOs "be assigned liability arising from requiring participating physicians to adhere to a specific set of clinical practice guidelines."

Thus, physicians are entrapped between MCO strategies for reducing the cost of medical services, which they must comply with in order to be compensated, and ethical and legal doctrines which hold them fully responsible and liable for patient harms arising from their failure to provide care of requisite quality. Even if they breach contractual requirements to follow practice guidelines in order to exercise independent judgement in the patient's best interests, they run the risk that if an injury results, the practice guidelines they ignored will be used by injured patients to show that such physician failed to meet the requisite standard of care. In such cases, physicians face liability unless they successfully refute this claim (Brennan, 1995). On the other hand, MCOs have virtually free rein to impose such pressures on physicians, and remain insulated from malpractice liability even if the pressures contributed to the patient's harm by constraining the physician from meeting professional standards.

Managed Care as a Source of Patient Safety

Like other organisations, MCOs practice risk management to prevent incidents which would cause them to incur economic loss, such as incidents which damage property, injure workers, cause disruption of activities, violate regulations or cause other harms for which they would be held responsible and bear liability.   Thus, MCO risk management involves the conventional process of

- identifying potential loss-causing incidents and estimating their likelihood and economic significance,
- prioritising the types of incidents according to their potential loss consequences,
- developing options for preventing the prioritised incident categories and for deflecting losses they would cause (e.g. insurance),
- selecting those options which are most cost-effective and compatible with the conduct of activities of requisite quality,
- implementing the selected options through internal procedures, training, performance incentives and other means and
- monitoring implementation practices and making necessary adjustments (Benda and Rozofsky, 1996).

Since full liability for harm to patients is usually imposed on physicians working for the MCO as independent contractors, as previously discussed, incidents involving medical error or malpractice do not receive high marks for risk prevention unless special circumstances will cause MCO losses. Among the special circumstances that could lead an MCO to prioritise such medical incidents are adverse publicity and notoriety which would damage the MCOs reputation and cause it to lose healthcare programme clients, particularly private healthcare programme clients that compete for patient subscribers. Other special circumstances involve incidents in some states (e.g. Texas) which have enacted legal reforms which enable injured patients to more readily impose malpractice liability on MCOs as well as physicians and occasional incidents arising from MCO fraud, misrepresentation or corporate negligence for which the MCO would incur liability in many states. (Stoekl, 1998).

Probably because medical error poses virtually negligible risk of economic loss to an MCO, except in the rare cases which have such special circumstances, MCO risk management is not seen as an effective means of preventing medical error. Instead, MCO practice guidelines imposed on physician contractors, and MCO screening and monitoring of physician contractors, are generally regarded as being more useful for assuring patient protection. Yet as previously discussed, practice guidelines are uncertain safeguards because they are designed to emphasise cost constraints on medical care, are not officially reviewed by disinterested experts, and in many instances, have not been developed or coordinated by physician organisations.

Screening and monitoring of physicians and MCO termination of those who are prone to committing injurious error may be more effective, but only after injurious incidents have accrued, and therefore does not fully serve the proactive, preventive purpose of risk management. In addition, MCOs review physician performance in terms of productivity, cost containment and other economic criteria and superior performance according to such economic metrics may outweigh inferior performance in providing non-injurious services, much as in industry where the production function often outweighs the safety function (Smith, 1997).

In addition, experience with risk management in medical contexts (e.g. hospitals) has shown that incident identification, evaluation and prioritisation are generally limited to past occurrences and fail to address foreseeable types of future incidents yet to be experienced, unlike industrial risk management. This means that medical risk management has not dealt with the consequences of change which can pose new risks: i.e. with potential for injurious medical error posed by introducing new diagnostic or therapeutic methods or instrumentation, by taking on new types of patients who have special conditions or needs, or by imposing new practice guidelines for use by physicians who have previously relied on other sources of knowledge (Benda and Rozofsky, 1996).

In addition, larger MCOs must deal with thousands of physician contractors and hundreds of thousands or millions of patients and encounter problems of scale in carrying out risk management procedures such as training, monitoring and coordination of multiple services. Finally, it is undeniable that the financial terms and practice controls imposed on physicians by MCOs are designed to reduce the costs of healthcare and do indeed cause many physicians to provide less than what they would otherwise do for patients. For these reasons, MCO risk management, practice guidelines and physician review procedures are insufficient for preventing injurious medical errors.

RELEVANCE OF CHEMICAL SAFETY MANAGEMENT EXPERIENCE

Experience in preventing injurious incidents, such as industrial accidents, in other business sectors could be instructive and help improve medical risk management. Some safety analysts have pointed to air traffic safety programmes as a source of learning that may be adaptable to the healthcare sector (Leape, 1994). Another business sector worth examining is the chemical process industry, where companies which make or use dangerous chemicals (e.g. toxic, reactive, flammable, etc.) have employed process safety management methods to prevent accidents, mitigate their consequences and respond to emergencies (Melhem and Stickles, 1997).

Chemical process safety management has, over time, become a rich mixture of facility design and standard operating procedures, sophisticated monitoring and control systems, human factors analysis and training programmes and self-auditing and organisational learning efforts. It must be compatible with company production and other business goals, assure compliance with regulatory requirements set by government agencies (such as the U.S. Occupational Safety and Health Administration and Environmental Protection Agency), satisfy the voluntary codes of conduct enacted by industry associations (such as the Chemical Manufacturers Association and the American Petroleum Institute), meet the standards of care established by the courts in order to avoid liability, implement safety measures set by casualty and liability insurers, and involve employees and host communities and be responsive to their safety concerns. (Baram, 1993; Baram, 1999; Stricoff and Baram, 1991).

However, efforts to learn from this decidedly different business sector face many obstacles. There are no definitive databases on chemical accidents and their causes, and no conclusive body of evidence establishing the value of a particular safety feature or type of safety programme for accident prevention. Compounding this uncertainty is the knowledge that many company-specific contextual circumstances, such as organisational and business factors, influence safety performance, but documentation is lacking. Nevertheless, some generic findings of a qualitative nature which provide lessons of potential value to healthcare management can be derived from review of chemical safety experience, as the following examples indicate.

Process safety management is not static, but varies from facility to facility, and also varies over time within each facility, due to changing business strategies and other dynamic contextual factors (such as organisational restructuring, market variations which affect revenues and the resources available for safety management, new productivity and profitability goals and competitive strategies, changes in regulatory requirements and agency enforcement strategies, and decisions to make or use new chemicals, to downsize and automate or hire independent contractors). Thus, organisational capacity to evaluate and manage risk under changing circumstances is difficult to develop but is necessary for maintaining process safety under real world conditions (Baram, 1999).

Despite improvements in process safety management, accidents are frequent. Company investigations to determine root causes have often been self-serving - usually implicating suppliers for equipment failure and workers for human error. More objective accident investigations by government agencies are now routinely conducted and increasingly find management failures – for example, not providing for a sufficient equipment maintenance programme or for employee training and emergency response, for eliminating safety margins due to cost and thereby causing facility design and operational procedures which do not forgive or tolerate foreseeable lapses by workers, for making decisions to operate beyond plant or workforce capacity, for downsizing the workforce and over-stressing the remaining employees, for failure to instruct and integrate independent contractors and part-time workers into safety management, for disregard of, or failure to learn from, near misses and not taking timely corrective actions. Thus, management inadequacies are now recognised as the ultimate root cause of many accidents. (Stricoff and Baram, 1991; Hale, 1997).

Many chemical plants are devoted to routine production of large volumes of a bulk commodity chemical (e.g. chlorine), and can easily standardise operations for optimal safety and efficiency. Others make single small batches of specialty chemicals and mixtures according to customer specifications and must frequently change production procedures without sufficient attention to the need for worker retraining or other necessary safety adjustments for various reasons (lack of time, resources or knowledge, for example) and therefore do not effectively standardise operations. As a result, such plants become reliant on their customers for safety information, which may not be reliable or adequate, to quickly develop *ad hoc* safety measures instead of systematic procedures carefully integrated into their plant and workforce. Thus, ability to successfully develop standard procedures is frustrated by the variability of risky activities as well as the time, cost and knowledge constraints involved (Baram, 1999).

Chemical firms, like MCOs, want to prevent incidents which pose unacceptable losses. Unlike MCOs, which are legally immune from malpractice responsibility and liability and face few losses of significance other than those arising from adverse publicity, chemical firms face the prospect of immediate major losses from chemical accidents. Such losses range from the destruction of plant, equipment, materials and other assets, to disruption of production and inability to serve customers, to tort and other liabilities for harms to property, workers and residents of the host community. Thus, the methods used for managing safety, and the vigour with which they are used, depend to a considerable extent on the loss consequences of mishaps (Stricoff and Baram, 1991; Baram *et al.*, 1992).

Government safety regulations and industrial safety codes provide a detailed set of organisational and management responsibilities for safety in the chemical process industry. Organisations must officially pronounce policy and commit resources in support of safety management. Managers must develop and implement accident prevention and emergency response programmes, establish procedures and train employees, document and audit practices to assure compliance, investigate and report violations, and communicate with labour, contractors and the general public on accident hazards and company safety measures. As a result, organisational and management accountability to regulators and industry associations has been established (North, 1997; Baram, 1999; Hale *et al.*, 1997). This contrasts with the absence of such requirements and management responsibilities in the healthcare sector. Thus, government regulators and industry associations can legitimate and facilitate the assumption of responsibilities for safety by organisational management and thereby promote the integration of safety and production functions.

Finally, chemical safety experts and industrial leaders have emphasised the importance of organisational learning from accidents and particularly from far more numerous near misses, so that timely corrective actions can be taken to continuously improve safety management programmes. The concept has been widely recognised by chemical firms and translated into procedures in many companies. However, experience indicates that actual practice is inadequate for several reasons: the difficulty of defining 'near miss', employee reluctance to report near misses due to fear of being implicated and blamed and unwillingness to implicate co-workers; management reluctance to receive reports of near misses due to liability exposure if corrective actions are not taken and an accident subsequently occurs; and management reluctance to investigate the causes of a near miss when this would disrupt production. Nevertheless, organisational learning programmes are growing, and several industry associations are attempting to promote inter-organisational learning by creating forums for companies to share the lessons they have learned from evaluating accidents and near misses. Thus fulfilling the promise of organisational learning requires careful preparation, incentives rather than punitive action to encourage reporting and evaluation of accidents and near misses and creation of an open, information-sharing company culture intent on continuous improvement (Hale *et al.*, 1997; Baram, 1999).

As this brief review indicates, some important lessons have been learned from chemical safety experience and merit further examination for possible adaptation and use in improving risk management in health programmes.

CONCLUSIONS

Effective prevention of injurious medical error in the context of aggressively managed health care will require a multifaceted strategy. Organisational culpability in causing physicians to depart from appropriate standards of care has been recognised and calls for official action to establish organisational accountability. Management practices for cost containment which require or induce physicians to provide inferior patient care need to be exposed and restricted. Standardisation in medical practice guidelines can conflict with physician judgement and the interests of the patient, and requires objective and expert review and coordination as well as physician capability to avoid compliance when medically necessary without financial retribution. In addition, health risk management deficiencies need to be identified and overcome by the introduction of lessons learned in other sectors of management experience, such as chemical process safety.

Thus, legal liability doctrines for medical malpractice should be extended to hold healthcare programmes and management intermediaries accountable for harm to patients caused by physician contractors when there is sufficient evidence to establish organisational culpability. This reform would internalise the social costs of managed healthcare by ensuring that liability would be proportionally allocated as appropriate between managers and their physician contractors. It could have the effect of causing MCOs or other management entities to refrain from imposing those cost constraints and practice guidelines which force physicians to provide inferior care, in order to avoid liability. In addition, MCO concern about such exposure to liability could give greater prominence to preventing medical error in their risk management programmes.

Although liability would have broad deterrent effects on health management, it has limitations, such as its dependence on costly litigation, the difficulty of proving organisational culpability and the availability of insurance to deflect liability from the organisation. Thus, reinforcement through government regulation and private self-regulation should be considered as methods of maintaining oversight and control over the cost containment measures imposed on physicians by health management organisations, thereby preventing measures which undermine the doctor-patient relationship and significantly interfere with the physician's ability to provide quality care to patients. Such regulatory and self-regulatory approaches could be patterned after those used to make management responsible for chemical process safety and would therefore be performance based rather than technically-detailed and prescriptive.

Standardisation in the form of medical practice guidelines needs expert and objective review and official certification and coordination. Creation of an independent board of physicians, public health experts and patient's interest representatives with authority to perform such functions and thereafter monitor approved guidelines and order their revision as appropriate, is called for. Authorisation of the board should provide that health programmes employ board-certified guidelines exclusively and that use of certified guidelines be conditioned on programme compliance with any requirements set by the board to assure proper use of the guidelines, such as the requirement that physicians and patients be allowed to depart from such guidelines when medically necessary without financial retribution or other sanctions. As with chemical process safety, official investigation of guideline-related injurious medical incidents for root causes and other research for the purpose of improving the quality of the guidelines, would be advisable.

Finally, healthcare programmes and their management intermediaries need to be stimulated to improve their voluntary efforts at medical risk management. Although exposing them to malpractice liability and regulation may provide sufficient stimulus, a more systematic and sustained effort aimed at educating medical risk managers about specific improvement opportunities and the benefits likely to be gained seems advisable. Lessons from chemical process safety, air traffic safety, and other risk management sectors could be presented for discussion and adaptation to fit the medical risk context.

'Best practices' from these other risk sectors would be particularly instructive and could involve presentation of methods for amplifying risk management to identify and address new risks posed by organisational change and other dynamic conditions, for doing self-evaluation of management inadequacies which contribute to risk, and for effectively implementing intra and inter organisational learning systems for continuous improvement (Lincoln, 1998). In addition, enlarging the scope of medical risk management by the incorporation of measures for responding to emergencies and mitigating the consequences of an injurious incident, subjects which have been neglected by health programmes, deserves attention because of proven value in industry.

Thus, principles of professional and organisational responsibility and practical lessons from risk management experience are combined to create this agenda for preventing medical error in the managed healthcare context. Pursuing the agenda may also serve an even more important societal interest, the need to maintain patient trust in physicians to provide quality care, the essential virtue of the physician-patient relationship which is now threatened by the complex medical enterprise created by managed healthcare.

REFERENCES

American Medical Association (1998). *Directory of Clinical Practice Guidelines*. Chicago.

Baram, M., P. Dillon and B. Ruffle (1992). *Managing Chemical Risks*. Lewis Publishing Co.

Baram, M. (1993). Industrial technology, chemical accidents, and social control. In: *Reliability and Safety in Hazardous Work Systems* (B.Wilpert and T. Qvale, eds.). L. Erlbaum Publishing Co., Hove, U.K.

Baram, M. (1999). Process safety management and the implications of organizational change. In: *Safety Management and the Challenge of Organizational Change* (A. Hale and M. Baram, eds.). Pergamon Publishing Co., London.

Benda, C. and F. Rozofsky (1996). *Managed Care and the Law: Liability and Risk Management, A Practical Guide*. Little, Brown and Co., Boston, MA.

Bovens, M. (1998). *The Quest for Responsibility*. Cambridge University Press, Cambridge, U.K.

Brennan, T. (1995). Methods for setting priorities for guidelines development: medical malpractice. In: *Setting Priorities for Clinical Practice Guidelines* (M. Field, ed.) pp. 99-110. National Academy Press, Washington, D.C.

Daniels, N. and J. Sabin (1998). The ethics of accountability in managed care reform. *Health Affairs Journal*, 17 (5), 50-64.

Furrow, B., T. Greaney, S. Johnson, T. Jost and R. Schwartz (1997). *Health Law*, 3d. ed. West Publishing Co., St. Paul., MN.

Hale, A., B. Wilpert and M. Freitag (eds.) (1997). *After the Event: From Accident to Organizational Learning*. Pergamon Publishing Co., N.Y., NY.

Hiepler, M. and B. Dunn (1998). Irreconcilable differences: Why the doctor-patient relationship is disintegrating at the hands of health maintenance organizations and Wall Street. *Pepperdine Law Review*, 25, 597-616.

Leape, L. (1994). Error in medicine. *Journal American Medical Association*, 272, 1851.

Lincoln, J. [1998]. *Environmental Health and Safety: Forum for Best Management Practices Manual*. Northeast Business Environmental Network, Lawrence, MA.

Melhem, G. and R. Stickles (1997). Engineering practice: enhancing safety through risk management. *Chemical Engineering,* 104, 20.

National Institute of Medicine (1995). *Setting Priorities for Clinical Practice Guidelines.* National Academy Press, Washington, D.C.

North, K. (1997). *Environmental Business Management,* 2d edition. International Labour Office. Geneva.

Robbins, D. (1998). *Managed Care on Trial.* McGraw-Hill Co., N.Y., NY.

Rochefort, D. (1998). The role of anecdotes in regulating managed care. H*ealth Affairs Journal,* 17(6), 142-149.

Sigma (1998). *Health Insurance in the United States: An Industry in Transition.* 2, 3-16, Swiss Reinsurance Co., Zurich.

Sisk, J. (1998). How are health care organizations using clinical guidelines? *Health Affairs Journal,* 17(5), 91-109.

Smith, T. (1997). Defining medical risk management metrics. *Preventive Law Reporter,* summer 1997, 19.

Stoeckl, A. (1998). Refusing to follow doctor's orders: Texas takes the first step in holding HMO's liable for bad medical decisions. *Northern Illinois University Law Review,* 18 (2), 387-409.

Stricoff, S. and M. Baram (1991). *Non-Regulatory Strategies for Preventing. Detecting and Correcting Accidental Releases of Hazardous Air Pollutants.* A.D. Little Co., Inc. Report to U.S. Environmental Protection Agency.

United States Law Week (1998*). States tell health plans that incentives may not limit medically necessary care.* Bureau of National Affairs, Inc., Washington, D.C., 67(15), 2227- 2228.

CHAPTER 14

APPROACHING SAFETY IN HEALTHCARE: FROM MEDICAL ERRORS TO HEALTHY ORGANISATIONS

Andrew Hale, Safety Science Group, Delft University of Technology, Delft, NL

The chapters in this book demonstrate the breadth and richness of the subject area of safety in medicine. Many themes can be distilled from them. I would like to concentrate on three:

- the nature of error in medicine and what are the productive and unproductive ways of considering it
- how we can best define, think about and achieve healthy organisations in healthcare, which have a high level of safety
- what sort of tools and methods we have and need to help us learn and achieve high levels of safety.

These themes are interwoven. The culture of organisations is partly determined by, and determines, the way in which people working in them think about errors and their preventability; only if errors are seen as preventable will people see the sense in trying to learn from them and develop tools to do so; the structure of organisations, or indeed of a whole inter-organisational sector such as medicine, determines the problems we shall meet in devising ways of communicating lessons across the boundaries, and hence the tools we need to do so. As an outsider to the medical world, these were the themes which came over to me as participant in the workshops, and after reading the chapters. In some aspects they show remarkable similarities with other technologies which have been more intensively studied; in other aspects they show clear differences because of the technology, organisation and, above all, the culture of healthcare.

IMAGES OF ERROR

Many of the contributions have stressed the fact that error in medicine is not easy to define. This is an insight that has grown over the years in many other areas of safety science (Leplat 1985). Even in the highly proceduralised world of the nuclear and chemical industry there is recognition that normative definitions of error are limited. They only capture the cases where there is one clear right way to carry out an activity which is agreed by the vast majority of practitioners. Where no one right way has been, or perhaps can be defined, the system is still in a state of learning. Only the result tells us whether the outcome of an action was successful or not, and then only about the result this time. Next time the same action, which saved a life this time, could contribute to ending one. This characteristic of the healthcare sector was often stressed in the chapters, particularly in respect of the more advanced surgical interventions, or in respect of new treatments tackling diseases which have been difficult to treat up to now. Medicine is, by definition, non-routine, is the claim.

This may be true of certain, indeed many, parts of the profession at certain times, but we should beware of letting this be an excuse for giving up the task of defining and agreeing on error altogether. Because not everything is black and white does not mean that everything is grey. All professions go through a stage in which they cloak themselves in the mystique of their skills and portray themselves as a brotherhood whose mysteries can only be learned by long apprenticeship absorbing the experience of the master. Skilled craftsmen in wood and metal trades did this in the 19th century, steelmakers and rubberworkers retained the arcane secrets of their mixtures and processes until the 1950s, designers still resist attempts to probe the thought processes and rules of thumb underlying their creativity. The medical professions have been among the most successful in resisting the advance of the protocol and have only embraced it fully in the last decade, and then not in all branches. However, where protocols are now established, this gives a starting point for characterising error. Even so, we need to accept the point, also frequently stressed, that healthcare remains an extremely complex activity where it is only possible up to a point to characterise patients, disease patterns and circumstances into categories which can be matched to accepted protocols. The scope for difference of opinion as to the correct course of action therefore remains large, but so too does the risk that an error of diagnosis will lead to the wrong choice being made. The pros and cons of the use of protocols and guidelines in improving safety and quality in healthcare will be an important research area for the future.

Central to any definition of error which is useful in the medical area must therefore always be the concept of expectation and consensus. Error is essentially something that the person who carried out the action must recognise for him or herself, because the result of the action was not what was expected. This is a useful definition as the basis for incident reporting and recording systems from which teams, departments and organisations can learn

(Koornneef and Kingston-Howlett, 1998) However, this is only a beginning. The figure of 4% cited by Staender *et al.* in Chapter 4, as the percentage of automatically recorded deviations which the team members considered worthy of reporting, should alert us to the fact that expectation is a problematic term in this profession. Several chapters emphasise that error or deviation seems to be equated with 'unrecovered' or 'uncommon' deviation. The image this conjures up is that medical intervention is seen as a race in which all that counts is finishing. The clinical imperative of life saving dominates. The slips, trips and falls along the way are so common and unremarkable that they are forgotten by the end and are not seen as interesting. Only if they are not recovered is it worth while learning from them. There is too much deviation in healthcare settings to spend time and attention worrying about all of it. Only when the 'mundane' business-related criteria of bed occupancy, medicine costs, patient satisfaction and comfort, re-operation and staff time are added to the success criteria of the establishment does the way the race is run become as important as the end result. Luckily there are increasing numbers of people and departments in healthcare who are paying increasing attention to such mundane criteria as the basis for their quality management programmes, on the back of which a number of the studies of safety reported here have ridden.

Any image is something which resides in the heads of people, and which is placed and retained there by the culture of the organisation and their experience of the reality of the environment in which they work. When the risks attached to medical interventions are intrinsically high, as in the case of seriously ill or injured patients, the contribution of manageable risk such as errors and hardware failures to the chance of survival can seem vanishingly small and hard work has to be put into keeping the pressure up for continuous improvement, however small that may be. Accidents as a cause of death in society in general have become much more visible in the last century partly because we have been so successful in controlling other causes of death such as infectious disease. Despite steady drops in the absolute numbers of accidental deaths, they have grown steadily in relative terms, particularly among the young and middle aged, as a cause of death. Hence they have gained more political and scientific attention. Hopefully this trend towards greater concern is already taking place, and will do so increasingly in healthcare, at least for the preventable accidents and incidents to otherwise young and healthy patients (such as the mothers giving birth in the study reported by Taylor-Adams and Vincent, Chapter 6). The more that safety can be seen as the prerequisite for pushing the limits of medicine further out, the more it will be seen as important even in the areas of the marginal patient.

Another aspect of the image of error, which is illustrated in the chapters on analysis of incidents, is the question as to which factors form the most important determinants of error and incidents. The overwhelming picture which emerges is that incidents in healthcare are seen as caused by human, and to a lesser extent, technical, failure. The step to a system-wide view of failure is a difficult one to make and is clearly still to be taken in many healthcare settings. The management and organisation of healthcare is still not placed centrally enough in the picture. In Chapter 13, Baram shows that it is a step which is actively resisted by the courts, at least in the USA. Jurisprudence still lays the most emphasis on the failure of the clinician and does not lightly shift the responsibility to the hospital which did not give enough time or resources. A move in this direction is essential if we are to make progress. In this light the introduction of concepts such as 'clinical governance' in the UK are welcomed, since they place the direct responsibility for the quality of care on the chief executive and not (just) on the individual clinician. Such a shift in thinking about liability has been made in other fields since the early 1980s, as the response to disasters such as Piper Alpha, Herald of Free Enterprise and rail disasters in the UK has shown (see e.g. Hale *et al.*, 1997). This has led to a much more systematic view of safety management and prevention. Powerful forces resist such a shift in health care, as Baram argues. Not least among them is the image which the medical professionals have of themselves. It is clear that doctors and nurses need to have a very high level of self-confidence in their own abilities in order to work in a profession which is so complex and where failure of their interventions is such a normal part of work. With such self-confidence it is easy for this to spill over into a belief that they can, and therefore should, control any situation that is thrown at them. Hence the pride in recovery from difficult situations; but also the deep concern about any discussion of fallibility. The analogy of the World War I or Battle of Britain fighter pilot, with his tales of the 'wizard prang' and 'flying by the seat of the pants', springs to mind. It is clear that there is much still to be done to tackle the image of error in the minds of all concerned in health, so that surgeons can feel comfortable stepping down from the pedestal on which society, but particularly the professional ethos and clinical training, have placed them. Only then can staff feel comfortable in openly discussing the issues of competence and motivation of themselves and their colleagues. In chapter 7, Carthey *et al.* show that this problem, also found in many other industries, is particularly great in healthcare. The rise of medical liability claims and the increasing readiness of patients to claim compensation works against more openness (e.g. Taylor Adams and Vincent – Chapter 6). The shift of liability from the individual to the corporate level may be the only way to create an oasis of trust within the organisation in which it can be openly discussed with sufficiently strong guarantees of individual immunity.

In order to capitalise on this medical culture of competence and pride in recovery, it is perhaps best that we emphasise two aspects of error:

1. Making errors and learning from them is the primary way in which we learn and build up competence; hence an open and constructive attitude to deviations is characteristic of a fully mature profession concerned about the quality of its work.

2. A second characteristic of a profession is that it knows its limits and does not claim to be able to exceed them; hence it is vital to recognise from incidents what were the preconditions outside one's control that set the stage for loss of control.

Putting these images together may help to encourage active discussion of deviations, and to encourage those concerned to identify the organisational factors underlying most of them. This points to the need to communicate across group and departmental boundaries, to influence earlier stages in the process, be that design and layout of equipment, or delivery of the patient or the resources from other parts of the system in the correct or expected state. This links patient safety very clearly to quality management.

As an aside at this point, it is perhaps interesting to note that every single contribution to this book, and to the workshop which led to it, is almost exclusively about patient safety. Only in Nyssen's chapter (3) is there mention of the fatigue and loss of motivation of the staff as something to be prevented in its own right. In other contributions such factors are only marginally present in so far as they are possible causes for errors by staff. In drawing analogies with other industries, this book is therefore essentially about quality management, where the quality of the health of the patient as the end product is analogous with the quality (and safety) of the car, chemical substance or foodstuff coming from the 'factories' of other technologies. We should ask ourselves whether this was just the chance composition of the workshop and those invited to attend, or whether it tells us something more essential about the way that safety fits into the medical culture. I would be inclined to think the latter. It is a culture of dedication to the patient, sometimes despite the cost to the medical staff in terms of overwork. It is therefore, perhaps, not surprising that the safety and occupational health of the staff receives little attention here.

APPROACHES TO SAFETY

Feeling the Edge, Not Following the Rules

Rasmussen's conceptualisation of the task of prevention, set out in Chapter 2, is an extremely useful one, which links clearly to the discussion on images of error. He sees the task of both the individual and the organisation as steering their activities through the sometimes well-known, but sometimes uncharted waters close to the edge. The edge is defined as the boundary at which unacceptable numbers of accidents, or an unrecoverable disaster will happen. The problem is that the edge, like the waters close to the rim of the flat earth in old beliefs, is shrouded in mist. He postulates that, in those waters close to the edge, there are untold riches to be found for those who dare. Implicit in such a picture of the task, if we accept the presumption that Rasmussen makes that there are always pressures pushing us closer to the edge, is that both individuals and organisations will always nibble away at margins of safety. Wilde describes this practice at the individual level as risk homeostasis (Wilde, 1994). Apart from Rasmussen's own examples of the same phenomenon, more are to be found at both levels in the later chapters in this book. Nyssen in Chapter 3 showed how the pressures to run tasks in parallel, or to anticipate actions rather than wait for clear signs before starting them, can narrow the margin to the edge. Others described the tendency, as intervention techniques get better and more successful (i.e. the margins tend to increase), to operate on sicker patients, and so to narrow them again. The practices of defensive medicine, mentioned by Baram, are attempts to plumb the waters near the rim in search of unsuspected reefs (or perhaps sharks in the form of ambulance-chasing lawyers), and so to widen the boundary of safety. This last is an example of the sort of recommendation Wilde comes to, of increasing the motivation to stay away from the edge, rather than shifting the edge further out by reducing the risk of any given action. The unfortunate thing is that this particular method of motivation results in high costs of unnecessary testing, which we must weigh against the positive benefits of increased care and supervision, better record keeping and communication with patients.

Rasmussen, and also Fahlbruch and Wilpert (Chapter 1), advocate a number of strategies and organisational characteristics as ways of steering a path which stays sufficiently back from the edge. The major one is to make the edge more tangible at all levels in the organisation, so that people can constantly feel it. Rasmussen warns against laying down detailed action rules, since these can lull people into the false sense of security that their actions are by definition safe. This can make them stop actively considering how close to the edge they are. This should not be seen as an argument against all attempts to make protocols, only as a warning about their form and their use. It always makes sense to have central repositories of knowledge about what are the best ways to handle in the wide range of circumstances which can be met. These are the memories of organisations and the body of knowledge of the profession. It would be a mistake to consider that these should be the rules which should guide everyday action. These operational rules need to be kept at a level that is not too detailed; no sub-clauses for every conceivable exception, but goals and considerations to be weighed for adapting performance.

One way, drawn from the findings of research on High Reliability Organisations (Rochlin 1989, Roberts 1989, 1990), to maintain the constant awareness of the edge and how to navigate along it, is to make the methods of work and the good and bad experiences of how things have gone into the constant topics of conversation of the team working on a given activity. In this way they are always alive, and an atmosphere of trust in each others' skills and openness is created. Mutual checking of actions can thrive in such an atmosphere, which provides an added group recovery mechanism for deviations. Contributions such as those by

Staender et al (Chapter 4) and Carthey *et al.* (Chapter 7) emphasised the importance of team work and openness in this way. The discussion of communication barriers and the tendency for healthcare systems to work in little isolated kingdoms, to be found in other chapters (e.g. Cromheeke - Chapter 10, Bogner - Chapter 5, see also Guldenmund and de Graaf, 1997), shows the negative side of this issue of openness to control and learning. The picture of the healthcare system to an outsider after reading these chapters may well be that it suffers some of the extreme forms of Taylorism. Taylor advocated, at the turn of the century, the sort of task division and specialisation which led to the assembly lines of the Ford motor plants. This specialisation produced spectacular productivity gains, but also led to feelings of alienation and loss of pride in achievement. Since the 1950s the manufacturing industries have been reversing that trend of sub-division and have been introducing job enrichment and task centred groups to restore meaning to work and to improve flexibility and communication. Healthcare still seems to be largely in the stage of skill- or discipline-based specialism. Activities are broken down into tasks given to completely separate individuals or groups. It is not at all clear who retains any overview of the whole process, or the whole patient, and communication is bureaucratised and de-personalised. The contribution of Büssing *et al.* (Chapter 9) is centred on this issue and describes it well, but leaves us still with the dilemma of how to cope with it. In a complex system, is it better to try to limit the communication need, by splitting the responsibilities more logically according to primary functional units, or to work on creating the circumstances for more active and easier communication between different professional and task groups? However we divide up tasks, we will create boundaries in one place as we remove them from another. The trick is to create active teams with high mutual trust in areas where the problems of risk control operate on a moment to moment basis (for example, an operating theatre) and to place the group boundaries at points where there is more time to work on effective communication. But then it has to be a high profile objective of the groups on both sides of that boundary to spend time on that communication.

Metaphors and Analogies

It was striking that the discussion at the workshop was full of metaphors and analogies. This chapter has used metaphors repeatedly to try to characterise different approaches to error and safety management. The metaphors which are used in talking about safety within an organisation, where people are seen as heroes and villains and the stories and myths which capture what we see as good and bad, are all manifestations of the culture of the organisation (Bolman and Deal, 1984). This can give insights into why safety is tackled in particular ways. What are, then, the useful analogies and metaphors for safety in hospitals?

Baram's contribution (Chapter 13) specifically raises the issue, present between the lines of many of the other contributions, as to what we can learn from a given industry to apply in another, such as hospitals, which have not yet been studied in depth. He uses the analogy with the chemical and nuclear industries, which have devoted the most time and energy so far in codifying safety management at all levels and in emphasising and specifying management responsibility. The models used in other chapters, such as those from Reason (1990, 1997) and van der Schaaf (1992) derive from the same industries, with additional insights from various transport activities, such as railways and airlines. These are all essentially bureaucratic organisations and the traditional metaphors of safety, which have been developed in them, emphasise the systematic, the rule-bound and the values of obedience and conformity. The nuclear and chemical industries have been strongly associated with such a centralised procedural-rational approach to safety, with its emphasis on predictability and planning and its link to the machine bureaucracy as organisational form (Mintzberg, 1979). Even in those industries this image has come under attack, as Rasmussen's chapter showed. The hospital certainly does not fit into such an analogy. It may aspire to be a rational professional bureaucracy, but the chapters, and more clearly the workshop discussions show that the reality is even looser. There is a large degree of improvisation constantly necessary, leading to the notion of an 'organisation on the run'. The hospital may be divided into fiefdoms often under the control of strong leaders and in a state of conflict, whether that is armed neutrality or even open war, with other parts of the system. It was notable that the physicians present at the workshop could all be characterised as mavericks, in the sense that they had defied the conventions of their professions by openly discussing and researching error and safety. This had been done at no small risk to their own reputations and was coupled with a high degree of competence and charisma to dare to break that mould. The metaphors which come more to mind than the systematic bureaucrat and careful manager, to describe the way in which doctors should be seen in the healthcare system, are those of the "very parfait gentil knight" (Chaucer - Canterbury Tales), or perhaps more the knights of the Round Table riding off into the forests (also places along the edge) to do battle for their high ideals and rescue maidens in distress (the patients) from evil dragons (risk and death). Such images of medieval knights imply also the shadow side of the romance, the compliant vassals and serfs who may not complain or speak out as equals to their masters.

In any case, the metaphors and analogies used in the workshop point to a much more confusing and conflictual situation as the reality of healthcare than is to be found in the machine bureaucracies of the process and energy industries. We need to be sure that the lessons we learn from other industries allow for that difference. Better analogies might be building sites, or primary industries such as agriculture, fisheries or mining. The difficult thing then is that we do not easily find such high performers in the safety field among those industries. If we are to draw lessons from petrochemicals, it would be more appropriate to consider exploration and production activities, with a high level of uncertainty from the environment, rather than refining or chemical production. Above all, this concern with appropriate analogies points to the need for the healthcare industry to learn from its own experience. In a careful study of how one's own industry works and how it arrives at its best achievements lie the best lessons for the future management of safety. From the failures we can learn too. The detailed case studies on which a number of the chapters of this book are based are therefore doubly welcome. It is to the issue of learning that I want to return in the last part of this chapter.

Learning How to Learn

The full complexity of risk management is revealed in looking at the healthcare system. It covers the whole life cycle of the patient, as we can see from the activities used as study focus in the chapters, from birth to degenerative and terminal diseases, such as heart failure and replacement. It also covers the whole life cycle of all the technical elements in the system, as Cromheeke's study of the heart valves (Chapter 10) showed, from manufacture, through use to failure. And, as that study and the chapter of van den Anker (Chapter 11) also show, the factors influencing the safety of patients reach well beyond the confines of the hospital or other healthcare institution into the lives of the patient before admission and after discharge. The range of system elements and interactions between them is therefore immense and the complexity of learning also.

The chapters can be divided into those which take the starting point of design or redesign and try to offer tools for making predictive assessments or rules for design, and those which concentrate more on the feedback side of the loop, by analysing current practice, or by collecting and trying to learn from incidents and accidents.

Of the former, Cromheeke (Chapter 10) presents life cycle analysis as a rational tool for making predictions about where to intervene, while Voges, in Chapter 12, places emphasis on system design rules in a normative approach. The study of de Graaf (1998), into the design of an intelligent anaesthesia monitor[1], used a combination of ergonomic approaches with a detailed study of the mental models of the eventual user, the anaesthetist, to arrive at an integrated design for supporting equipment. His starting point is that we must fully understand how the anaesthetists currently conceptualise their tasks and the state of their patients, if we are to build equipment which supports that task - a participative ergonomics standpoint. All these are rational, predictive, system-based tools which have great potential in specific areas.

---

[1] presented at the workshop but not included in this book

If there is one thing that shines through as a major difference between the chemical and nuclear industries and the healthcare system, this is the attitude to technical innovation. The former industries see the potential of technology as a solution to many safety problems, but have exceptionally stringent change management systems in place to assess any technological changes for their potential hidden dangers of undermining well established safety systems. The attitude to new technology in healthcare seems much more reminiscent of the car driver or fishing boat owner (Stoop, 1990) keen to lay their hands as fast as possible on the latest technical advance, cram their vehicle (or operating theatre) full of it and try it out. New technology seeps into the system at all levels, based on decisions by many independent people (often the consultants) and with comparatively little assessment of its system-wide impact. Perhaps this is one instance where tighter control, based on rational, systematic predictive tools for design could be taken over from the process industries. At least technology needs to be questioned, particularly the introduction of new technology, much more than it currently is.

The need to think in advance about the implications of change may be satisfied in other ways, though. The chapter of van den Anker and Lichtveld (Chapter 11) fits into this idea and makes an interesting contrast with the rational, deductive methods, in that it aims to devise a tool to help designers of new systems to visualise their consequences better. It does not aim to come up with logical predictions from the method itself, but to stimulate the people in the system to articulate their expert knowledge about how things work and might change. In this way it involves the user in the design process and in the safety of the solutions for the whole system.

We can see a similar dichotomy in the methods aimed at feedback. The field studies (Nyssen, Carthey *et al.*, Büssing *et al.*, Staender *et al.*) all used triangulation of data from a number of different sources. Some, such as incident recording and categorisation systems, are aimed at producing rational and hopefully complete classifications of failures and elements which could be changed. This pushes us to closed-ended, pre-classified lists to be filled in with ticks and crosses. However, the studies always complete the picture with rich descriptive data on a small number of incidents, which put flesh on the rather dry bones of the rational methods. These can only be collected with open-ended, free report methods, through participant observation or in-depth interview.

This contrast points to two different ways of thinking about learning. One is learning seen as the rational accumulation of knowledge in systematic categories, followed by prioritisation based on (semi-)quantitative reasoning and then rational improvement. This fits the structural rational image discussed in the last section. Contrasted with this is the more holistic 'aha-erlebnis', where the incident or situation triggers the imagination and, above all, acts on the motivation to improve matters. The actual improvement may not necessarily be drawn directly from the incident, which may not be appropriate to the circumstances or needs of the learner at that moment, but may be inspired by it, or drawn from his or her own knowledge, triggered by the rich text of the description or visualisation. A similar contrast has been suggested between the value of systematic, but dry, standards or rules for solving health and safety problems, and the richer but often less directly applicable data found from reading actual solutions applied in practice and the experience of what were good and bad aspects of them (see, for instance,. Hale and Swuste, 1997).

Underlying a consideration of what are the best sources of data for learning is the question as to what is sufficient proof for making changes in the way things are done. With the increasing move to evidence-based medicine, there is increasing pressure for a higher level of proof of the need for and efficacy of safety improvements. This will drive the need for better and richer incident reporting and analysis systems in order to point the finger at the crucial determinants. However, we should be wary of too great a shift in this direction. There is ample evidence (e.g. van der Schaaf *et al.*, 1991; Hale *et al.*, 1997) that safety reporting systems are very vulnerable to any attempt to use their data for proving blame. As soon as this happens, there is an incentive either to stop reporting, or to bias the coding to prove the point that the reporter or analyst may want to make. We should not lose sight of the value of the rich incident report used not for scientific proof, but for stimulating action.

Any study in this field needs to combine both types of data and to realise their biases when combining them to produce a clear picture for learning. Self-reporting and free, rich incident data are open to bias through the sort of images which were discussed in the first section of this chapter, but they are much more real and motivating to the user. Quantitative, closed-end reporting, either automatic from a simulator or direct monitoring instrument, or from standardised reporting systems can be much more objective, but does not live and breathe in the same way. Above all it is vital that those who are going to need to do the learning and changing are directly involved in setting up the data collection system, collecting and interpreting the data. Otherwise they will have no ownership of it and will see learning as something to be done by others and not them.

CONCLUSION

It is clear from reading these chapters that we have a long way to go in meeting the challenge of making healthcare safer. The appearance of this book is a step in the right direction. Its very existence attacks the taboo around talking about error and subjecting it to detailed study. Hopefully it 'decriminalises' the concept in the eyes of those who need to do the talking, namely the doctors who are in positions of power in the organisation, and who have, up to now, had the most to lose 'culturally' from such openness. Hopefully, it will also raise the profile of the debate about the potential conflict between the movement towards more medical liability claims and the move to make the prevention and management of safety more explicit and open. Patients must have the right to compensation for injury caused by poor safety management, but we must find ways of achieving this which do not drive the errors and failures which cause the injuries underground. Only with open debate can learning take place, and this is one of the main defining characteristics of a healthy organisation.

Fahlbruch and Wilpert (Chapter 1) list the following characteristics of organisations with good safety records:

1. A sense of mission
2. High technical competence and performance
3. Structural flexibility, with redundancy in loosely coupled situations and close coordination in tightly coupled ones
4. A combination of hierarchical and team authority with the different means of communication appropriate to each, so as to cope with both loose- and tight-coupled situations
5. Continuous improvement as goal
6. Rewards for error discovery
7. A culture of reliability
8. Continuous training

In addition they argue for

9. A system-wide perspective and model of safety, with
10. Good feed-forward and feedback learning systems.

From the chapters of this book and the discussion above it would appear that healthcare establishments generally score well on criteria 1, 2, 5, 7, 8. They always have been placed with a clear vision and mission to save life and increase health. That mission is defended in all the debates around state regulation or privatisation and has been the rallying cry of the medical professions to resist what they see as the insidious encroachment of business thinking and cost-benefit analysis. Without wishing to attack the central importance of this mission, I hope it is clear from my discussion that I think it needs some nuances building into it in order to allow not only patient safety, but also staff health and safety a clear place. The valiant knight racing to rescue the damsel in distress needs to take the time to tighten the girth, check the quality of the shoeing of his horse and think about whether the design of his helmet enables him to see the potholes in the road he is charging down[2].

The level of competence and technical support to be found in healthcare is also impressive. This too needs to be the basis from which all attempts to improve safety set off. It would be a fatal mistake to imply that safety measures are a vote of no confidence in the

---

[2] Or perhaps he delegates this to his horse.

skills of staff. What has to be promoted is the view that the sum of all those individual competences has to be supplemented by better adaptation of the individual and the technology to each other, and above all, by the development of real function-based team work in which all contributions are equally valued and add up to more than the sum of the parts.

Continuous improvement is also an increasingly explicit goal of healthcare, as is concern with a culture of reliability. Quality management programmes have been introduced in many countries into the hospital sector, which have made performance measures a much more acceptable and accepted concept. The professionalism which underpins the mission of healthcare also places improvement as a personal goal. As this book has shown, it is possible to attach the goal of increased patient safety to this motor of care quality improvement, but only if we can succeed in making safety as measurable as other outcomes of care.

Finally, on the positive side of the equation, continuous training is also an integral part of the world of healthcare. The hierarchy of posts, the integration of formal training and experience-based learning and the central place of research in the medical professions make learning at the individual level a central good. I have argued above that we need to build on this by adding the organisational level of learning, based on better incident and accident analysis and the promulgation of the idea that there is an important level of organisational responsibility over and above the individual one. The acceptance of such an addition is one of the largest challenges for the healthcare industry.

On the negative side, or, if we wish to make this more positive, the challenges for the industry are in finding the right balance between criteria 3 and 4 and in creating the complex of criterion 6 with criteria 9 and 10. There is a very strong hierarchy in healthcare, with the doctors on the top level and nurses and other groups further down, with conflict over the place of the administrators. We have seen that communication can suffer considerably under this regime. At the level of the direct patient care there are often much more flexible practices, which belie this hierarchy, but it is clear that much more research needs to be done to study explicitly what are the best structures and relationships for different parts of the health care system. Team work has been emphasised greatly in the chapters and warrants still more study to determine how it can be optimised, particularly across discipline groups. It is an open question as to the degree that groups and communication can be redesigned on functional grounds, rather than on discipline grounds. A central theme in any such research will be the degree to which, and the way in which, certain parts of healthcare can be subjected to more protocols, guidelines and care plans. The value of these is that they make expectations explicit about how care should be given and what the 'errors' or deviations are which should be reported and studied. The danger of them is that they suppress creativity and active coping and promulgate an attitude of rule following. The optimal course between Scylla and Charybdis will be a matter of careful experimentation and research.

Perhaps the largest question mark rests over the image of error and safety in health care. Only gradually is it becoming acceptable to discuss and research error in clinical settings. There is a long way to go before staff will be rewarded and promoted on the basis of the openness with which they talk about and learn from their errors. I suggested earlier that one path to this is to try to link learning from errors into the complex of the image of professionalism and continuous learning which is central to the medical professions. Steps in this direction are case discussions on 'the incident of the week' from which the whole l team, and eventually the whole organisation, can learn (Koornneef, personal communication). Such discussions need to emphasise not only the changes which the team itself can make, so increasing their professionalism, but also the factors which lie outside their control and which need to be communicated actively with other parts of the organisation. This can hopefully increase the realisation that individuals' performance is conditioned and limited by the way the organisation operates, the resources provided, the quality of interdepartmental communication and information exchange, and the way in which successive parts of the organisation are equipped to respond to changes, crises or problems in other departments. Only if that can be achieved, will the image of error as an individual problem gradually give way to the system-wide perspective and model of safety which Fahlbruch and Wilpert advocate.

The book provides some promising lines for advance, but it falls far short of solving many of the problems that Rasmussen indicates in his chapter. One of the most difficult of those is how to make the edge of safe performance tangible for the managers who allocate the time and resources and who create the many detailed situations in which error and accidents are facilitated. This is a problem which healthcare shares with all other industries, and which will occupy the research community and the aware manager for many years to come. Lurking behind the discussions in this chapter is a still more fundamental question, namely the degree to which the technology and the current organisational structure of health care provide the opportunity necessary to change the safety culture. How much more safely can we manage care without having to change things like contractual relationships, departmental structures, communication and information technology? Again this is a question which is occupying safety managers and researchers in all industries (Hale and Hovden, 1998). Change is endemic to all technology and organisation, but we know too little as yet about how such change can drive safety, or indeed how explicit requirements for more safety can and should drive change.

REFERENCES

Bolman, L. G. and T. E. Deal (1984). *Modern approaches to understanding and managing organizations*. Jossey-Bass. San Francisco.

de Graaf, P. (1998). *How to design an intelligent anaesthesia monitor: safety and cognition based design in anaesthesia monitoring*. Doctoral thesis. Delft University of Technology.

Guldenmund, F. and P. de Graaf (1997). *AMC-ISA project: nulmeting (Base line measurement)*. Safety Science group. Delft University of Technology. Internal report.

Hale, A. R. and J. Hovden (1998). Management and culture: the third age of safety. In: *Occupational Injury: risk, prevention and intervention* (A.-M. Feyer and A. Williamson, eds.), pp. 129-166.Taylor & Francis. London.

Hale, A. R. and P. Swuste (1997). Avoiding square wheels: international experience in sharing solutions. *Safety Science*, **25** (1-3) 3-14.

Hale, A. R., B. Wilpert and M. Freitag (eds.) (1997). *After the event: from accident to organisational learning*. Pergamon. London.

Koornneef, F. and J. Kingston-Howlett Accident data in organisational learning, or what makes accident databases useful? In: *Accident databases as management tool* (E. de Rademaker and J-P. Pineau, eds.), pp.171-184. TI-KVIV. Antwerp.

Leplat, J. (1985). *Erreur humaine, fiabilité, humaine dans le travail.* (Human error and human reliability at work). A. Colin, Paris.

Mintzberg, H. (1979). *The Structuring of Organizations*. Englewood Cliffs: Prentice Hall.

Reason, J. T. (1990). *Human error*. Cambridge University Press. Cambridge.

Reason, J. T. (1997). *Managing the risks of organisational accidents*. Aldershot. Ashgate,

Roberts, K. H. (1989). New challenges in high reliability research: high reliability organisations. *Industrial Crisis Quarterly*. **3**. 111-125.

Roberts, K. (1990). Some characteristics of one type of high reliability in organisation. *Organisation Science*. **1**(2). 160-176.

Rochlin, G. I. (1989). Informal organisational networking as a crisis-avoidance strategy: US naval flight operations as a case study. *Industrial Crisis Quarterly*. **3**(2). 159-176.

Stoop, J. (1990). *Safety and the design process*. Doctoral thesis. Delft University of Technology.

van der Schaaf, T. W., D. A. Lucas and A. R. Hale (eds.) (1991*). Near miss reporting as a safety tool*. Butterworth-Heineman. Oxford.

van der Schaaf, T. W. (1992*). Near miss reporting in the chemical process industry. Doctoral thesis*. Technical University of Eindhoven.

Wilde, G. J. S. (1994). *Target Risk*. PDE Publications Toronto.

NAME INDEX

SUBJECT INDEX (by chapter number)

Lightning Source UK Ltd.
Milton Keynes UK
08 September 2010
159601UK00001B/23/P